Remaining Relevant

Remaining Relevant

Achieving Lifelong Professional Success

Karen Lawson, PhD

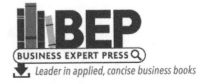

Leader in applied, concise business books

First published in 2022 by
Business Expert Press, LLC
222 East 46th Street, New York, NY 10017
www.businessexpertpress.com

ISBN-13: 978-1-63742-252-6 (paperback)
ISBN-13: 978-1-63742-253-3 (e-book)

Business Expert Press Business Career Development Collection

First edition: 2022

10 9 8 7 6 5 4 3 2 1

To my husband, Robert Lawson, for his love and support
and
To my mother, Mildred Eells, who, by example,
instilled in me two valuable character traits—resilience and perseverance

Description

Motivated by necessity or simply desire, many people are remaining in the workplace well beyond the traditional retirement age. According to the Bureau of Labor Statistics, in 2026, the percentage of workers aged 65 to 74 is projected to be more than 30 percent, up from 17.5 percent in 1996. This is supported by a 2018 survey conducted by the Transamerica Center for Retirement Studies. Half of the 6,372 workers polled don't expect to retire at 65, and 13 percent plan never to retire. Furthermore, according to the World Bank, the average life expectancy in the United States is 78. That translates into more people who can and want to remain in the workforce. However, in our growing youth-centric environment, baby boomers (born 1946–1964) and traditionalists (born 1922–1945) often feel marginalized, dismissed, and even invisible. This book offers practical tips to help baby boomers and traditionalists remain significant, credible, and relevant in today's work world.

The target audience includes men and women who are still actively engaged in their chosen professions or who have started new careers. It is a *how to* for those who want to overcome ageism as part of the anti-retirement movement.

The content is based on research as well as interviews with men and women from a variety of professions including finance, real estate, manu-facturing, marketing, law, and medicine, to name a few.

The book also includes self-assessments, checklists, and activities read-ers can use to create action plans for those areas they would like to target for continued self-development.

Keywords

relevance; reinvention; ageism; age bias; career transition; revitalize; semi-retirement; anti-retirement

Contents

Endorsements

"Yes, Virginia, there is a work life after 65! Karen Lawson's newest book, Remaining Relevant, *is the 21st century's primer for the traditionalist and baby boomer generations who aren't ready to retire at 65 but face issues of ageism and relevance in the workplace. After losing a long-standing business client who told Lawson her material and information were not relevant, the author has written a book full of relevant material and information. Lawson offers personal and practical advice, from 'Don't Retire' to 'Reinvent Yourself' with everything in between. Based on her many years as an internationally recognized consultant specializing in organization and management development, and executive coaching, Lawson's book is a must read for anyone over 65 and who wants to stay active and find relevance in the working world."*—**James Mundy, Historian, The Union League Legacy Foundation**

"After reading the Preface, Introduction, and first two chapters, frankly, I am hooked. Karen Lawson's Remaining Relevant *provides an inspirational playbook on growing older without getting old. Passion and purpose are her guiding lights, supported by specific practical suggestions on actively compensating for the inevitable aging process. I enjoyed reading the book and will be personally guided by many of her suggestions."*—**Peter S. Longstreth, President, Consular Corps Association of Philadelphia**

"As a Gerontologist, I am excited for Dr. Lawson's book to hit the press. Ageism is still embedded strongly in our American culture. Dr. Lawson's book is a great call out to those of us in the workplace to prevent ageism and reject stereotypes and assumptions through her sage advice. Multigenerational workplaces are key to success to stay relevant to all customers. Dr. Lawson provides excellent advice on how to engage with different generations—so we can be best able to contribute and navigate new environments."—**Karen Kent, PhD, Director, MBA Program, DeSales University**

"Karen Lawson tackles the sensitive and rarely broached subjects of ageism and relevance in a thorough and unique way. I am one of those people who never plans to retire, and while I am not yet feeling that disjoint with a younger professional generation, I plan to deploy some of the broad array of practical tips and exercises found in this book to ensure it stays that way. I particularly appreciate the various communication and voice tips regarding vocal fitness and word usage, emphasizing the advice, 'Don't let your language date you.' Remaining Relevant *should be a must-read for those who see no sunset in their career journey and want to remain successful along the way."*
—Marynell Benson, Healthcare Executive; Board President, Providence Animal Center

"Karen Lawson hits a home run with her new book Remaining Relevant: Achieving Lifelong Professional Success. *Based on her years as a consultant, speaker, and author, she outlines eight very practical and concise tips to turn retirement on its head. Her personal account of a client who deemed her irrelevant spurred the writing of this book. Some of the topics Karen focuses on include staying sharp and connected, seeking harmony, and keeping up with technology. The best parts of the book are the self-assessments, checklists, and activities that help you outline your own plans for self-development. Rest assured you will gain greater insights regarding your own relevancy, and you will unquestionably want to share this with friends and colleagues who are facing similar challenges."*—**Kim McConnell, President, McConnell Leadership Group**

"Remaining Relevant *provides information that is helpful for people of all ages in our society.*

I couldn't put the book down. Every page was truly relevant to me and my experiences in the workplace and in life in general. I work in a very young industry where being in your 40s or 50s makes you the Senior person in the room. I've been on the receiving end of ageist tactics or comments made by upper management that Karen Lawson cites in her book. I've found all the insights and strategies Karen discusses in her book to be exceptionally beneficial.

This book would be very helpful not only to those over the age of 50 but also for junior and middle management employees to read as part of employee training so that they can better understand how to positively interact with, motivate, and learn from employees in their company who may be older and/ or who have more seniority than they. I highly recommend everyone read Remaining Relevant.*"*—**Sue Laks, Founder, Real Media Fusion, LLC**

"As we reach retirement age, some of us decide to pursue day-long leisure without responsibility. Others elect to continue to pursue their professions or decide to use what they have learned during their careers and professionally engage the world in a new way. Karen Lawson's book, Remaining Relevant: Achieving Lifelong Professional Success *is more than a guide to those of us who don't view retirement as an end. Lawson's book is also an important guide to keeping relevant and effective during the many years we pursue our professions.*

Author Neil Pasricha cites a study of the people of Okinawa where there is no concept of retirement from work. Life is a continuum, where people move through life's phases. Pasricha writes, 'They don't even have a word for ... [retirement]. [Their lexicon] has the word "ikigai," (pronounced "icky guy"), which roughly translates to "The reason you wake up in the morning." It's the thing that drives you the most.' It is their reason for being.

Having a reason to wake up in the morning, remaining relevant, and being successful at what you do is a key to a successful life. Lawson's book points the way."—**Stan Silverman, Founder and CEO, Silverman Leadership**

"Dr. Lawson's thorough research on being relevant is clearly evident in the first paragraph of Chapter 1. The book is laid out in a useful way incorporating meaningful exercises to solidify learning and comprehension of challenging topics. Her knowledge and expertise as an educator are evident; this book is useful and impactful."—**Cindy Wollman, Berkshire Hathaway Home Services, Fox Roach**

*"*Remaining Relevant *is a must read for anyone who is feeling their age and/ or experiencing any age discrimination in their career. This book is a useful reference guide, full of practical nuggets for reinventing yourself and staying current in our ever-changing work landscape."*—**Marilyn Manning, PhD, CSP, CMC, Owner of The Consulting Team, a management consulting firm in Silicon Valley, CA**

"Remaining Relevant *is a must-read for baby boomers and traditionalists who wish to remain in the work environment past retirement age. Dr. Lawson gives helpful tips on how the post-60-year-old employees can be relevant, significant, and credible in today's world. Dr. Lawson also offers useful self-assessment tools to create an action plan for self-development and reinvention. I find this book a perfect how to as I transition from a 35-year career with the Federal Government into a new profession working with animals. Thank you, Dr. Lawson.*"—**Karen Refsnyder, Animal Alternative Healing**

Preface

Motivated by necessity or simply desire, many people are remaining in the workplace well beyond the traditional retirement age. According to the Bureau of Labor Statistics, in 2026, the percentage of workers ages 65 to 74 is projected to be more than 30 percent and those age 75-plus almost 11 percent. However, in our growing youth-centric environment, baby boomers (1946–1964) and traditionalists (1922–1945) often feel marginalized, dismissed, and even invisible. This book, *Remaining Relevant,* offers practical tips to help baby boomers and traditionalists remain significant, credible, and relevant in today's work world. These tips address areas such as physical appearance, communication, health, technology, relationships, and mental agility.

The content is based on research as well as interviews with dozens of men and women in their 60s, 70s, and 80s who are still actively engaged in their chosen professions or who have started new careers later in life. Their backgrounds include finance, real estate, marketing, law, manufacturing, medicine, and consultancy. Some own their own businesses while others are employed by firms or corporate entities. I also interviewed professionals such as health care professionals and image consultants who offered their expert opinions on many of the topics in the book. Another group of people who provided valuable insight were millennials (1979–1997). To them, I posed one simple question: "What do people in their 60s, 70s, or 80s do or say that make them seem old to you?"

Many of the points or suggestions I make in this book may not apply to you because either you are already practicing the behaviors, or they don't suit your personal style or preferences. As you read some tips, you might think, "I already know this!" That is probably true—nothing you haven't read or heard before. The key questions, however, are, "Are you actually doing it?" or "Are you doing it consistently?" As the Stage Manager in Thornton Wilder's play *Our Town* says, "There are things we know but we don't take them out and look at them very often."

Sometimes, we just need to be reminded. So, I hope you will take away not only some reminders but perhaps some new *ahas* as well.

Why this book and why now? There are many books and articles on the market that focus on preparing for retirement or making your retirement years meaningful and productive. To me, those publications inadvertently create an either-or situation: you are either retired or planning to retire. What about those who are neither? Many older people in today's workforce have no intention of retiring. When I asked those I interviewed, "When are you going to retire?" all but one person said, "Never." Taking the response a step further, Dennis Powell, owner of Massey Powell, a public affairs consultancy, said, "When I stop thinking." Professional speaker and humorist, Allen Klein's response about retirement was quite emphatic: "Never! I need to accomplish what I want to for as long as I can."

Despite our desire and determination to continue working, unfortunately, many baby boomers and traditionalists are forced to retire (due to company policy) or are sidelined. Sidelining doesn't happen suddenly. More often than not, it's gradual and insidious. In case you're wondering if you are being sidelined, consider the following indicators:

- Excluded from important meetings
- Omitted from the distribution list of key communication pieces
- Passed over for promotions
- Prime clients or projects given to younger colleagues
- Not being offered training opportunities

As many people pointed out in my interviews, ageism is alive and well. No longer is age valued in the workplace as it once was. Older employees used to be revered for their experience, wisdom, and knowledge. In some companies and professions, this is still true. For example, in some professions such as law and medicine, age and experience are still valued and respected. As Lloyd Remick, a top-rated entertainment and sports attorney in Philadelphia, Pennsylvania, now in his 80s shared with me, young associates seek him out to *pick his brain* because they look up to him and value his experience. When courting potential young clients, Lloyd takes them on a tour of his offices where the many platinum and gold records of his clients adorn the walls. As he related to me, "By the time they get to the conference room, they're sold. Age is not an issue. Experience and success say it all."

Far too often, however, age is perceived negatively. Older workers are regarded as *over-the-hill*, not *with it*, resistant to change, stuck in the past, and lacking energy. This became quite apparent to me when I turned 70. The first incident happened on my birthday when I went for lab work prior to a doctor's appointment. Upon reviewing my paperwork, the technician said, "Happy Birthday. You don't look 70." Of course, I wanted to say, "What is 70 supposed to look like?" To this day, I still get these questions: "Are you still working?" or "When are you going to retire?" The most impactful interaction came when I contacted the president of a company for whom I had been conducting leadership development programs for the past 12 years. I called her in December to get the schedule for my sessions starting the following month.

Me: "Hi. It's that time of year again, and I'm calling to get the schedule for our training sessions starting in January."

Client: "Oh, I'm sorry. I meant to call you. We have decided not to use your services going forward."

Me: "Of course, I'm very disappointed but can you tell me your reason and who you are going to use instead?"

Client: "I won't tell you who we have engaged because it hasn't been finalized yet. I will tell you that the reason we are no longer going to use your consulting services is because your material and information are not relevant."

Me: "This is the first time I have heard about this. Can you give me some examples?"

Client: "No, I really can't. It's just some general feedback I have received."

Me: (after more attempts to uncover specifics) "I appreciate your candor, and I do hope you will keep me in mind for future opportunities."

As you might imagine, I was quite upset and even shed some tears. I really felt useless, defeated, and old, especially after I learned that the consultant they engaged to replace me was in her early 40s. Although that incident was devastating, it was a turning point for me and served as the catalyst for this book.

What does *remaining relevant* mean? I began each of my interviews with that question, and as you might expect, the responses were quite diverse. However, certain words and phrases stood out: participate, contribute, adapt, useful. Although the words were different, they seemed to underscore the theme of adding value and being valued. These sentiments expressed by the people I interviewed were summarized quite eloquently by Geoffrey James in his article "4 Ways to Become More Relevant" for Inc.com: "In the business world, to be relevant means being an integral part of your organization, of your company, of the economy, and of the future. It means being the kind of person on whom others depend, whether for leadership, expertise, acumen, or emotional support."

The perception that older people are no longer relevant is reinforced by the terms *elderly* or *geriatric* when referring to the over-65 set. This is in stark contrast to some parts of Japan that have banned the use of *elderly* for anyone under 75. Instead, people who are in the 65–74 range are to be called *pre-old*.

The insights presented in *Remaining Relevant* will show you how to overcome stereotypes and perceptions to help you remain a valuable professional contributor regardless of age.

My philosophy is that I can't do anything about getting older, but I can do something about getting old. Growing older is about the natural aging process. Although we can't stop it, we can slow it down. Growing old, however, is another matter. Growing old involves mind, body, and spirit, which I will address throughout the book.

Acknowledgments

I am deeply grateful to the following men and women who generously contributed their time and shared their experiences and expertise to make this book a reality: Katie Barrett, Dr. Robert Brookman, Rosemary Browne, Phil Bruschi, Dr. Gayle Carson, Birtan Collier, Major General (retd.) Wesley Craig, Rosa Cucchia, Melissa Davey, Dr. Gary Dorshimer, Paul Dougherty, Bob Fischer, Paul Heintz, Casey Johnson, Allen Klein, Linda Knox, Pepper Krach, Leo Levinson, Brian Lipstein, Thomas J. Lynch, William Maston, Dennis Powell, Lloyd Remick, Bobby Rydell, Mitchell Sargen, Dianne Semingson, Gregory West, James Wilson, Jr., and Cindy Wollman.

A special thank you goes to Vilma Barr, Collections Editor for Business Expert Press, who has encouraged and guided me along the way. Her insights have been invaluable.

Introduction

Don't Retire

The trouble is when a number—your age—becomes your identity,
you've given away your power to choose your future.
                    —Haruki Murakami, Japanese Writer

About Retirement

When people ask me when I'm going to retire, my response is "Never! It's not in my vocabulary." Most people are shocked. In fact, I have had people in their 40s tell me they can't wait to retire and wonder what's wrong with me.

Fueled by consumerism and an aging population, insurance companies, financial planners, the media, and retirement communities divide our lives into preretirement and postretirement. The premise for this book is don't retire. Here's why. Traditionally, *to retire* is to leave one's job or cease to work, typically upon reaching a certain age. Interestingly, the origin of retire is from the French *retirer* meaning *to withdraw* or *retreat* to a place of privacy, shelter, or seclusion. Most people who retire in today's world view retirement quite differently. They see it as an opportunity to relax, wind down, pursue interests and activities they were not able to do when they were working full time. However, there are many of us who do not plan on retiring.

Although the points in this book can apply to people at any age, *Remaining Relevant* is written for people who are still actively engaged in their professions or careers. A career is broadly defined as a lifelong endeavor that you work toward every day. It can include several jobs and/ or employers and involves education, work experience, training, and purpose beyond just working for a paycheck. A career is also fueled by passion for the work you do. For example, I am passionate about and have built a career as an educator. Within that career, I have had many jobs such as high school English teacher, college professor, corporate training director, consultant, author, professional speaker, and executive coach.

Changes, Challenges, and Choices

It was spring 1988, and I was invited to deliver the commencement address at the high school from which I had graduated. I thought long and hard about the title and theme for my speech, and finally decided on "Changes, Challenges, and Choices." I don't remember much of what I said that day, but that same theme popped into my head as I began writing *Remaining Relevant.* We may not be starting out, but we share much in common with graduating high-school seniors as we embark on the next phase of our lives and careers. We are once again faced with many changes, challenges, and choices.

Changes include our health, finances, career, status in the community, relationships with family and friends, interests, and lifestyle. These changes create *challenges,* and the *choices* we make to overcome or mitigate them is key to our remaining relevant. Yes, we can choose how to meet those challenges. I often hear people say, "I don't have any choice" when faced with a challenging situation. My response is, "You always have a choice." Sometimes the choice is an action; sometimes it's a psychological or emotional response; sometimes, it's both. For example, when my client told me she was no longer going to use my services, I was flooded with emotion—anger, hurt, disbelief. My initial reaction was defensiveness and then defeatism, resignation, and acceptance. Negative messages swirled in my head: "I'm too old," "Nobody wants me," "I'm washed up," "I have nothing to offer." After wallowing in self-pity for a while, I chose to take action by first taking stock of what I had to offer and how I could leverage my experience and expertise in a new way. Then I developed an action plan to reinvent myself. This book is one of the action items in my plan.

Ageism is insidious and the last acceptable bias. We can overcome ageism, not by complaining to human resources, protesting, or filing lawsuits. We can take action to remain on top of our career game by adapting, remaining flexible, and making changes in ourselves. We may not be able to eradicate ageism, but we can influence others not to engage in it by taking charge of our behavior, attitudes, and mindset. My client did me a favor. At least she had the courage to say what many think.

To me, retirement is a state of mind. Researchers have found that when people believe they can do it, a concept known as self-efficacy, they perform better. This power of positive thinking can work wonders. It's your choice to let your age define you. You can do remarkable things at any age. Here are some examples:

- Giuseppe Verdi was still composing operas in his 80s.
- Oliver Wendall Holmes was still dominating the Supreme Court until he retired at 91.
- Leopold Stokowski recorded 20 albums in his 90s and signed a six-year contract at 96.
- Betty White, with the longest television career of any female entertainer, was still performing well into her 90s.
- Gladys Burrill ran a marathon at 92.
- Dorothy Davenhill Hirsch went to the North Pole at 89.
- Mary Higgins Clark, author of over 50 successful suspense novels, was still writing at 90.
- Frank Gehry, noted architect, designed new galleries and public spaces for the renovation of the Philadelphia Museum of Art at 91.
- Florence Rigney, America's oldest working nurse, retired from a Tacoma, Washington hospital at 96.
- Iris Apfel, fashion icon and businesswoman, was still modeling at age 100.
- Betty Reid Soskin became a park ranger at age 84 and is the National Park Service's oldest active member at 100 (as of this writing).

Before we can take action to make others see us as relevant, we must first see ourselves as relevant. Sometimes it seems easier just to give up and let things happen—*que sera sera,* whatever will be will be. That's the easy way out. This book is about not giving in or giving up; it's about resilience, perseverance, and relevance.

Retire or don't retire. It's your choice.

CHAPTER 1

Stay Sharp

Exercise your mind the same as you would exercise your body.
Practice healthy habits that will help you, empower you, and
improve your perspective.

—Akiroq Brost, Author

Does this sound familiar? You walk into a room in your home, stop, and say to yourself, "What did I come in here for?" Or perhaps you can relate to some or all of the following:

- "What's the name of that restaurant we like?"
- "Where did I put my car keys?"
- "It's on the tip of my tongue."
- "Lately I have such a hard time remembering names."
- "I think I'm having a senior moment."

Don't despair. You're not *losing it*, and you're not alone. You may dismiss or accept these incidents as simply part of the aging process. However, brain functions need not decline with age. The challenge is to delay or slow down the rate of decline. The key is to accept normal age-related changes and actively compensate for them. Maybe you will need to put a basket or hook by the door to the garage as the place you put your car keys so that you won't misplace them. Perhaps you could keep a *little black book* where you jot down the restaurants you have frequented and your own mini reviews to help you remember your favorite ones.

Brain Research

Although recent research suggests that some aspects and processes change as people get older, simple behavior changes can help people stay sharp for as long as possible. The inevitable physical changes in the brain produce behavior changes. Some people have difficulty finding the words they want. Others have to work harder planning and organizing their activities. As we age, neurogenesis (the birth of brain cells called neurons) slows down in our hippocampus, the part of the brain that plays a major role in learning and memory. The good news is that we can increase neurogenesis through exercise and mental stimulation. What does decline is episodic memory, our ability to recall specific events that happen to us such as where we parked the car at the mall.

A group of researchers led by Michael Marsiske, associate professor of clinical and health psychology at the University of Florida, found that short mental workouts improved performance and was sustained even five years later. For example, learn a new language or learn to play a new musical instrument. These types of activities can be helpful in preventing memory problems or developing dementia or Alzheimer's. Take advantage of free online language-learning platforms such as Duolingo or Memrise, offering dozens of different language courses. Personally, I'm working on French and spend 15 to 20 minutes a day on a lesson.

Memory Fitness

Perhaps you remember the phrase, "The mind is a terrible thing to waste." Coined by the advertising agency, Young and Rubicam, over 40 years ago to promote the United Negro College Fund scholarship program for Black students, this slogan can easily be applied to those who just stop exercising their minds. To stay sharp, you must keep your mind active.

Mental acuity or sharpness involves memory focus, concentration, and understanding. It's an indication of how well your mind is working. Continually challenge yourself with new experiences and learning new things. One thing you should *never* do is to complain about memory loss. If you say you can't remember things, it becomes a self-fulfilling prophecy because we act on our beliefs.

Howard Gardner, author of *Frames of Mind,* supports the contention that the mind must be challenged. According to Gardner, "The mind is like a muscle. If it is constantly challenged with learning, it grows stronger; if not, it weakens." Offering further support of the importance of keeping your brain active, Phil Bruschi, author of *Mind Aerobics: The*

FundaMENTALSs of Memory Fitness, points out that "exercising your brain strengthens your mental abilities, just as exercising your body makes your muscles stronger."

As noted earlier, not all types of memory decline with age. Our capacity to recall knowledge learned even at a young age stays with us throughout our lives. If you have any doubt, play *Trivial Pursuit* or watch *Jeopardy!* As a regular viewer of *Jeopardy!*, I am amazed and quite pleased by how many answers I get correct from my sofa. Seemingly useless and irrelevant pieces of information I learned in school or acquired from experience during my lifetime just pop into my head.

The following assessment is a modification of the original "Your Memory Profile" developed by Phil Bruschi. Its purpose is to provide feedback regarding your behaviors, beliefs, and attitudes regarding memory fitness and those that need improvement. Place a check mark beside the statements that apply to you most of the time. Be as candid as possible.

1. I seek out opportunities to learn and challenge my mind as I grow older.
2. I watch television game shows such as *Jeopardy!* and *Wheel of Fortune.*
3. I look for ways to stimulate my mind, personally and professionally.
4. I watch educational television programs.
5. I am open-minded to trying memory techniques, even if they seem silly or illogical.
6. I play games that exercise my mind, such as crossword puzzles, Scrabble, Sudoku, chess, and brain teasers.
7. I look for ways to improve my memory skills.
8. I read detective or mystery books.
9. I try to remember information by picturing it in my mind.

Look at those items that you checked. Consider those you did not check and use them as a basis for your self-improvement plan.

Many people believe and accept that the older you get, the more difficult it is to develop one's memory. This just isn't so. Memory is a learned skill, and there are steps you can take to improve or enhance your memory. Before we address ways to increase your memory fitness, let's look at two types of memory—short term and long term.

Short-term memory (or working memory) is the capacity for holding a small amount of information in an active, available state for a brief period. This working memory—the center of conscious thinking—has an estimated capacity of six to nine *chunks* or pieces of information. The information in your short-term memory will be forgotten within about 10 seconds unless it is repeated over and over, or it is transferred to long-term memory.

Long-term memory can hold millions and millions of separate bits of information over the course of a lifetime. To improve your memory, you need to increase your ability to transfer information from your short- to long-term memory. To help us remember, we need to be able to retrieve information out of our long-term memory into the conscious state of short-term memory. As we age, it does become more difficult to recall information, especially short-term memory.

When we are unable or find difficult to recall information stored in long-term memory, it's easy to blame it on aging; however, there may be other factors that can interfere with memory. Consider the following potential barriers:

1. Poor listening skills
2. Mind wandering
3. Distractions
4. Lack of interest
5. Stress
6. Physical pain
7. Lack of sleep
8. Fatigue
9. Information overload

There are many actions you can take and practices you can incorporate into your life to improve your memory.

Memory Devices

Mnemonics

Mnemonics are memory aids based on association. Two such strategies are *acrostics* and *acronyms*. An *acronym* is an abbreviation made from the first letters of the words in a sequence. For example, ASAP stands for As Soon As Possible. Another example comes from my childhood piano lessons. To learn lines of the treble clef (EGBDF), my piano teacher taught me to recall the phrase, Every Good Boy Does Fine. I remember it to this day, many years later! Isn't that so much easier to remember than five unrelated letters? On the other hand, an *acrostic* is a piece of writing in which the first letter, syllable, or words of each line spells out a word. I have created several acrostic job aids for my training programs. Following is an example of one I developed for conflict resolution:

Resolving Conflict

Respect the other person's position or point of view.
Empathize by "putting yourself in the other person's shoes."
State your position clearly and unemotionally.
Own your role in the conflict.
Listen actively to the other person.
Value the relationship.
Engage in mutual problem-solving.

Notice that the letters that begin each guideline form the key word to dealing with conflict: RESOLVE.

Chaining and Pegging

Both *chaining (linking)* and pegging employ *visualization*.

Visualization is the mind's ability to picture an event or item. Chaining is associating one thought to another. As Phil Bruschi puts it, "When you want to remember a new piece of information, it must be associated or 'linked' to something you already know in some illogical way. This technique uses visual imagery to associate two or more items for remembering lists of things in sequential order." Guidelines for chaining are as follows:

- Select the items you want to remember.
- Create a story using the words you want to remember.
- Make the story absurd to associate the items.

- The items can be larger or smaller than they really are, or they can be objects in action.
- Put yourself in the story.

Here is an example:

I want to remember the following words in sequential order: shoes, book, dumbbell, pumpkin, fan, glasses, flag, candle, towel. After my workout, I visualized myself sitting on a pile of *shoes*. I wanted to read a *book* so I used a *dumbbell* to smash a nearby *pumpkin*. Inside I found a *fan* that I used to cool off. To help me relax, I used my *glasses* in the shape of a *flag* to light a *candle*. I covered myself with a *towel* and fell asleep.

The second technique that uses imagination and association is pegging. Pegging uses visual imagery to associate anything you need to remember with images previously associated with numbers. Numbers are abstract, so to make them more concrete, you need to hang these new items on established images. A simplistic example that I use around the Christmas holidays is when I try to remember the song, "The Twelve Days of Christmas." I picture these items as I go through each of the days:

1st—Partridge in a pear tree
2nd—Two turtle doves
3rd—Three French hens
4th—Four calling birds
5th—Five golden rings
6th—Six geese a-laying
7th—Seven swans a-swimming
8th—Eight maids a-milking
9th—Nine ladies dancing
10th—Ten lords a-leaping
11th—Eleven pipers piping
12th—Twelve drummers drumming

Observation

Seeing and observing are not the same.

- Seeing is a complex process involving various parts of the eye that results in signals being sent to the brain, which then interprets them as visual images.
- On the other hand, observing goes beyond the process of capturing and interpreting what the eye *sees*. Observing involves using all our senses and the brain analyzing data it receives from the sensory information transmitted. To enhance your observation skills, try the following activity:

Leave the room you are in, preferably one that is not familiar to you. From another location, describe the room you were in with as much detail as possible. Include chairs, lamps, wall ornaments, flooring, curtains, blinds, number of windows, location of furniture, other accessories, and even smells and room temperature. Now return to the room and compare your written description with the actual scene.

When I was a bank training director, we used the following activity to help new tellers understand the importance of keen observation. During the middle of a teller training class, we had a stranger come into the room to talk to the trainer. When the visitor left the room, the trainer asked each of the trainees to write down a description of the visitor and what they saw and heard. Not surprisingly, each person had a different description.

Have a System

The key is to accept the normal age-related changes and actively compensate for them. There are many tools available today to help you manage your daily life. If you have trouble remembering what you need to do, try these tips:

- Make daily *to do* lists. It doesn't matter what system you use—an old-fashioned paper-based system or something more high tech. There are plenty of apps for your smartphone. You just need to find the one that works for you and follow it.

- Jot down notes. One of the people I interviewed keeps a very small *little black book*, which he uses to write down things he wants to remember about people such as a characteristic or their favorite restaurant, television program, color. Another one of my interviewees adds details or pieces of information about someone to the person's profile using her smartphone.

Keep Your Mind Active

Just as you need to incorporate physical strength training into your daily life, you also need to strengthen your mental muscle. It is critical to keep your mind active even as it relates to small, seemingly insignificant behaviors. For example, do you or someone you know have a habit of asking others to "remind me to…?" This is not a behavior you want to practice if you want to stay mentally fit. First, asking people to remind you to do something is abdicating responsibility and putting the onus on others for your behavior. Besides, what happens if the person you asked doesn't remind you? Is it his or her fault if you don't take action? You are clearly not exercising your brain by turning that responsibility over to someone else. I'm not suggesting that you try to remember everything you need to do. In the spirit of the Chinese proverb, "The palest ink is better than the best memory," write it down. *Make a list*, electronically or the old-fashioned written *to do* list aforementioned. Set a time on your mobile device or laptop to remind you to pick up the dry cleaning, take your pills, or call a client.

Keep Up With Trends in Your Industry

Every profession and industry is experiencing rapid change, and if you don't keep up with the trends in your industry, you will be left behind. Attend professional conventions and conferences. It's easy to say to yourself, "I've been going to these conferences for 30 or 40 years, and I know all this stuff. These events seem to be for the younger folks who are building their careers. I've been there, done that."

The truth of the matter is that because things are changing so rapidly (especially technology), you can't afford not to go. Not only are you going to learn about new trends through the formal sessions, but you will also gain a wealth of knowledge just by interacting with people who are younger than you. As public relations and advertising expert, Leo Levinson, owner of GroupLevinson Public Relations, puts it, "The real danger to those of us who are more seasoned is to come across as being out of touch."

You should spend two to three hours a week on professional development. That could take the form of reading professional publications in your field, attending meetings of professional organizations, or participating in seminars or webinars. Professional speaker, entrepreneur, and savvy businesswoman, Dr. Gayle Carson, made it a point to participate in two seminars or webinars a month. At age 83, she showed no signs of slowing down until she lost her long battle with breast cancer.

Play Games

Crossword puzzles, Sudoku, Wordle, brain teasers, and strategy games are helpful in forming and retaining cognitive associations. Play online brain games. Brain games are games or activities that can help assess and train your mind, your brain, and your cognitive skills. Examples are CogniFit, Peak, Elevate, Mensa Brain Training, and Luminosity. These programs offer a free trial period and then encourage you to sign up for their subscription. AARP has a program called Staying Sharp that is included in your membership or can be purchased without joining the organization. In addition to brain games, Staying Sharp offers articles, activities, recipes, and videos related to brain fitness. Even watching (and, of course, playing along) game shows such as *Jeopardy!* and *Wheel of Fortune* can challenge your brain.

Become a News "Junkie"

An effective way to remain relevant is to keep up with what is going on not just in your own country but the rest of the world. Make a conscious effort to seek information from a variety of news sources—not just those that reflect your own political beliefs. Make sure you are exposing yourself to both liberal and conservative viewpoints. Employ various formats such as broadcast and print. Access a variety of news resources, both network and cable.

Read—A Lot

I already mentioned the importance of reading publications related to your field, but you need to read other types of publications and topics as well. Read mystery and detective novels to exercise your memory and powers of observation. Also, find out what your clients and younger colleagues are reading so you can engage in conversations during social interactions.

Get Involved

Most likely, as a successful professional, you are already involved—maybe even too involved. However, fight the tendency to slow down or drop out. Continue to seek opportunities to volunteer your time and talents in professional organizations and community groups. Start a mentoring program to help others who are just starting their careers. For example, the Forum of Executive Women in Philadelphia sponsors a mentoring program designed to enhance the leadership skills of emerging women leaders in the community. The program involves monthly Mentoring Circles in which mentees and mentors discuss a variety of topics related to leadership. During the 10-month period, forum members meet with their assigned mentees and provide guidance on career goals, personal and career development, and workplace relationships.

Go Back to School

I can remember thinking about and wanting to go back to school to earn my doctorate. I was 44 at the time and was afraid that I had been out of college so long that I wouldn't be able to succeed. I mentioned my concerns to a friend and said, "I'm going to be 50 years old by the time I get the degree." She responded, "You're going to be 50 anyway. So do you want to be 50 with or without the PhD?" Her words made so much sense. I did enroll in the doctoral program and received my degree at age 49.

Throughout the five years I was in the program, I was inspired by the other students many of whom were my age or older. In fact, one woman who became a close friend as well as a colleague in the training field was 70 when she finished the program.

Learn Something New

Research has shown that people who continue to learn new things are less likely to develop Alzheimer's disease or dementia. As Vilma Barr, collections editor for Business Expert Press puts it, "Keep learning is the key to non-retirement." If you are not interested in doing something formal like working on a degree, just enroll in courses that might interest you. Many colleges and universities offer interesting online and classroom-based courses for the over-55 crowd. In addition to academic resources, you can sign up for online courses offered by professional associations and online course providers such as Coursera. Harvard Online Courses are even free.

Engaging in learning activities that are entirely new and have nothing to do with your work is not only stimulating but also makes you a more interesting, well-rounded person. If you live in large metropolitan areas such as New York, Philadelphia, or Boston (among others), it's likely you have One Day University. As the name implies, the program's one-day sessions feature four or five lectures by leading university professors from prestigious colleges and universities. They also offer hundreds of archived and live-streamed lectures on a variety of topics.

Another example of course offerings that people can take just for the fun of it is the Osher Lifelong Learning Institute (OLLI) of the University of Delaware. They offer courses in the arts, humanities, information technology, languages, math, and sciences. A membership cooperative for adults over 50, the program "provides opportunities for intellectual development, cultural stimulation, personal growth and social interaction." Some of the more interesting topics include "One Act Operas," "Investing for a Successful Retirement," "Interviewing Movie Stars," "A History of Wine," "Genealogy: Fundamentals of Research," just to name a few. The only downside to this particular program is that courses are offered during the day; however, there are many colleges and universities that do offer evening courses.

Watch Educational Shows

Incorporate shows that make you think and help you learn new things into your weekly schedule. Great sources are PBS specials and the Discovery Channel.

Teach Classes

Teach a course at a local community college or lifelong learning program. Check their offerings and see where your topic would fit. The topic could be related to either your vocation or avocation. Many local colleges and universities have robust and varied lifelong learning continuing education programs and would love to add someone with your background and experience to their faculty. A major benefit to you is that you would be learning from and interacting with people of different ages and from different backgrounds. You would remain relevant out of necessity.

Dr. Gary Dorshimer continues to teach Fellows in Sports Medicine at the University of Pennsylvania in addition to his private practice and serving as team physician for the Philadelphia Flyers professional hockey team. Dr. Dorshimer says that "teaching keeps me relevant because I have to keep up with what is going on in my profession. The people I'm teaching are reading and learning every day and expect me to have the answers to their questions." At the same time, Dr. Dorshimer stresses the importance of "knowing the basics and how to adapt them and apply them to current situations."

Become a Thought Leader

When you see or hear the term *thought leader*, several questions may come to mind. What is a thought leader? Why is it important to be regarded as a thought leader? How do I become a thought leader? Let's take these one at a time.

A *thought leader* is generally considered an expert in his or her field or industry. He or she is the *go-to* person, that is, the trusted resource or adviser who not only has the experience and expertise in a certain area but who is also innovative and dedicated to developing others to follow in their footsteps and create a foundation for others to build on or to join.

Becoming a thought leader is important because it helps you increase your visibility and worth. Being regarded as a thought leader gives you exposure and access to people who make things happen in your organization or community. People will want to connect with you because you are regarded as someone who is *in the know* and respected by your peers. In many cases, being known as a thought leader will open doors to seats on corporate boards, industry committees, and promotions within your organization. It can also create opportunities to gain national and even international recognition.

Not everyone can become a thought leader, and you can't just say, "I am a thought leader," and expect others to seek you out. People are declared thought leaders by someone else. Those third-party endorsements come from others' experiences with you. To be recognized (or regarded) as a thought leader, you must become known for your cutting-edge practices, innovative thinking, and change leadership. You become a person who influences the thoughts, attitudes, and behavior of others.

Chances are you are already a thought leader and don't even know it. Your experience, knowledge, expertise, and credibility you have demonstrated over the past several decades have established you as the person others turn to for information, inspiration, and insight. Your challenge is to leverage your background and experience and have others recognize you in that role. Being known as a thought leader doesn't happen overnight. It takes time, knowledge, and expertise in a certain field or profession.

Don't Overlook the Mind–Body Connection

The mind–body connection is powerful at any age, but its impact and significance as we age becomes even more important. Regular aerobic exercise has been shown to aid cognition by boosting blood flow, which brings more oxygen to the brain. Mental acuity or fitness is impacted by nutrition and diet. Research shows that certain food can enhance or hinder one's ability to concentrate and remember. According to a study published in JAMA (*Journal of the American Medical Association*), people in their 70s who walk three times a week decrease their chances of developing dementia by 30 percent.

A healthy diet is also essential for a better memory. The Mediterranean diet, a plant-based style of eating, is highly recommended for both mental and physical health. The diet is a simple combination of fruits, vegetables, fish, whole grains, nuts, beans and peas, and olive oil. These foods are rich in memory-enhancing nutrients and low in saturated fat. Furthermore, fatty fish such as salmon, tuna, anchovies, and sardines, among others, provide Omega 3 fatty acids proven to improve overall health. Finally, the antioxidants found in berries, citrus fruit, apples, and dark chocolate benefit our health by preventing or slowing damage to cells in our bodies caused by environmental and other stressors.

We will discuss more about physical fitness and nutrition in Chapter 5, "Get Physical."

Take Action!

- Enroll in a course (online or in person) that is not related to your career or profession.
- Start playing a game that challenges your mind.
- Teach a continuing education course (fee or free) at your local high school, community college, or online course provider.

CHAPTER 2

Communicate Clearly

Communication—the human connection—is the key to personal and career success.
—Paul J. Meyer, Founder, Leadership Motivation, Inc.

You may be wondering why this chapter is even in the book. After all, by the time you have reached this point in your career, you have pretty much proven you know how to communicate. Right? Well, not quite. Although you have been a successful communicator thus far, I'm sure you agree that communication has changed a great deal. And I'm not just talking about the technology involved with communication or the variety of methods and modes of communication. We will address those in more detail in Chapter 7, "Keep Up With Technology."

In this chapter, we will focus specifically how your approach to communication can make you relevant or irrelevant in today's world. *Communication is the most fundamental, complex, and critical human interaction, and it is becoming more so.* Communication, although never easy, was at least simpler. Business was conducted primarily through face-to-face meetings and telephone conversations. Then along came e-mail and, for the most part, we learned to accept that as part of business communication as well. Things, however, began to get complicated with the introduction of social media, chat, and instant messaging.

In his book, *Silent Messages*, Professor Albert Mehrabian of UCLA shares results of his study dealing with the relationship among the three elements present every time we are engaged in a one-on-one, face-to-face interaction. The study, however, only relates to communication involving feelings and attitudes. According to Mehrabian, each communication is a transaction made up of the following:

- Verbal   what we say (words)
- Vocal   how we say it (tone)
- Visual   how we show it (facial expressions, body language)

For us to be believable, there must be consistency among these three elements. These elements must be congruent. Interestingly, the element that has the greatest influence is visual with 55 percent, followed by vocal (38 percent). What we actually say (verbal) accounts for only 7 percent! That does not mean that our words are not important. Rather it underscores that people will believe what they see more than what they hear.

Delivering Your Message: Verbal

Words matter. They can be helpful or hurtful; informative or insidious; instructive or destructive. We influence and are influenced by words. Once spoken or written, they cannot be taken back, and they can be retrieved. Just ask anyone whose past has come back to haunt them. Many leaders (think government official, company CEO, and so forth) have been hurt and their careers ruined because of poor word choices. As colleagues, parents, and friends, we often use words and phrases that either encourage or discourage, without knowing the impact or results of our remarks.

The adage, *think before you speak,* is so applicable, especially in today's environment. Because words are both powerful and fragile and can be easily misinterpreted, it is important to choose the right words to convey your message or express your feelings. Have you ever been in a situation when you made a statement, the person to whom you were speaking reacted entirely differently from what you expected? Choose your words carefully. As Mark Twain once said, "The difference between the almost right word and the right word is really a large matter—'tis the difference between the lightning-bug and the lightning."

Look at the following *discourager* phrases and check those you might be guilty of using:

- *Yes, but...*
- *We've tried that before and...*
- *What you mean is...*

- *Let's discuss it some other time...*
- *You have to...*
- *I don't have time right now...*
- *It's not in the budget*
- *Why did you...?*
- *That's a dumb idea...*
- *You don't understand...*
- *You're wrong about...*
- *You're over-reacting...*

How did you do? Many of us are unaware of the impact of these phrases and others like them on other people. You might be thinking about now, "Well, I may use these phrases sometimes, but I really don't mean them to be negative." That may be true; however, the next time you are tempted to use a *discourager* phrase, ask yourself the following questions: What is my intent? How am I (or would be) perceived? Remember, perception is reality.

Read the following list and notice how much more positive and encouraging these phrases are. Think about the impact of this list versus the preceding list.

- *That's an interesting point...*
- *I appreciate your hard work...*
- *I never thought of that...*
- *I have faith in you...*
- *I know you can do it...*
- *You're on the right track...*

Can you think of others to add to either list? If you find yourself using any of the *discourager* phrases, reword the phrase to be more encouraging and positive.

Using "I Messages"

I messages are statements designed to give the receiver feedback about his or her behavior. The use of *I messages* promotes open communication. They are very effective in reducing the other person's defensiveness and resistance to further communication. The responsibility lies with the sender who delivers the message honestly, expressing feelings, focusing on behavior description, not evaluation.

On the other hand, *you messages* blame, accuse, or attack the other person, causing him or her to respond emotionally and negatively. Because an *I message* communicates how the sender experiences the other person's behavior, the receiver is more likely to accept the sender's comments as positive feedback. As a result, the receiver will respond more positively.

This is particularly important when giving feedback to our younger colleagues, who do not react well to what they perceive as negative feedback. Keep in mind that the millennials, in particular, were brought up receiving awards for just participating and hearing *good job*, regardless of whether it was a good job or not.

Giving Directions or Instructions

How many times in both your personal and professional life have you given someone directions or instructions? You may have given someone directions to your house or simply told a person what you wanted him or her to do. Then when the other person doesn't do it *right*, that is, according to your expectations, you naturally blame the other person for not listening. Always keep in mind that what may be perfectly clear to you is not always clear to the other person. Although giving directions should be a two-way process, the onus is on the sender of the information to make sure what he or she meant is what is received and understood. Someone once said, "I know you believe you understand what you think I just said, but I'm not sure you realize that what you heard is not what I meant."

Delivering Your Message: Vocal

No matter how old we are, we can still improve our ability to deliver our messages orally. This is even more critical as we age. Like it or not, younger people (and sometimes even our peers) make judgments and assumptions about our capabilities based on our voice. As we age, our voices may become weaker, harsher, louder, and so forth, depending on our physical health as well as our gender. From about age 65, male voices become higher and tremulous, whereas women's voices get deeper or remain the same. Many who are experiencing a hearing loss tend to talk louder. Not only can this label you as old, but it can affect overall vocal health.

As we age, our vocal cords weaken and become drier and *stringy*, which prevents normal vibration, causing higher pitch voices that sound thin. This is particularly true for men. Although vocal changes are a natural part of aging, these changes can affect others' perception of you as well as your self-perception.

Although voice changes are a normal part of aging, there are things you can do to keep from sounding old. Just as you engage in physical exercise to keep your muscles in shape, you must do the same with your voice. Below are some strategies you can use to improve your vocal fitness:

- *Drink more water.* We have all heard about the benefits of drinking a lot of water throughout the day from aiding weight loss to improving skin tone, as noted in more detail in Chapter 5, "Get Physical." People, however, don't think about how important water is to our voices. Although vocal cords are not directly touched by the fluids, they are lubricated by a fluid made by nearby glands. This will not happen if the body is not kept hydrated.
- *Sing.* If you have a good voice, consider joining a choir at your place of worship or perhaps through a community organization. If that isn't your skill set, sing along to the radio or iTunes in the car on your way to work (if you're alone) or sing in the shower. If you sing in the shower, the benefits are twofold. First, you are exercising your vocal cords, and second, the steam from the shower will lubricate your voice box. Be careful, however, not to strain your voice by singing too loudly.
- *Read out loud.* Reading out loud keeps your voice working and provides it with the exercise it needs to stay healthy. Read a newspaper or magazine article out loud to yourself, spouse, or even your pet. Take advantage of opportunities to read to your grandchildren. Another idea is to seek out community programs that welcome volunteers to read to children or

community centers. You will benefit from the vocal exercise, and those to whom you are reading will benefit from the experience.

- *Don't strain your voice.* You must care for your vocal cords (muscles) the same as you would the other muscles in your body. This means, don't shout. If you work in an occupation that is noisy and requires you to shout to be heard, you need to rest your voice every five minutes.
- *Avoid spicy food.* Spicy food can cause acid reflux that irritates and dries out the throat.
- *Don't smoke.* Smoking dries the inside of the larynx and scars the vocal cords, resulting in a raspy voice.
- *Take care of your throat.* If you have a cold with laryngitis or a cough, you will need to take extra care to rest your voice to prevent scarring. Over-the-counter medication can certainly help, but seeing your doctor is preferred.
- *Improve your posture.* Not only is good posture important in helping you look young, it is also essential in keeping your voice young. Slumping prevents deep breathing and causes your vocal cords to work harder. Exercises, such as Pilates, are a great way to strengthen your core that results in better airflow.

We have all heard the phrase, "It's not what you say but how you say it." Your tone of voice communicates volumes. We convey our emotions through how we express ourselves. Tone of voice also clarifies meaning and impacts how people perceive us, relate to us, and may determine whether they are willing to listen to us. In many cases, our tone contradicts the words we say. To illustrate how tone of voice can impact meaning, say the word *no* to express different emotions and meanings:

No. (firm refusal)
No! (surprise)
No. (disbelief)
No? (questioning)
Nooo. (sarcasm)
No. (reprimand)

Try this exercise to reinforce the importance tone and inflection. Then think about when someone misinterpreted your intent because of the way you said it. Say each of the following statements out loud, emphasizing the word that appears in bold and think about how the meaning changes depending on the word emphasized.

I never said she didn't like you.
*I **never** said she didn't like you.*
*I never **said** she didn't like you.*
*I never said **she** didn't like you.*
*I never said she **didn't** like you.*
*I never said she didn't **like** you.*
*I never said she didn't like **you.***

Delivering Your Message: Visual

As mentioned earlier, nonverbal communication or kinesis has a profound impact on our interpersonal interactions. Our body language reveals our true emotions and feelings and thus reinforces or contradicts what we say. Furthermore, our nonverbal behaviors send strong messages that contribute to people's perception of us.

Posture

Not only is posture an important part of nonverbal communication, but it also plays an important role in our physical health, as discussed in Chapter 5, "Get Physical." Standing tall and sitting up straight communicate confidence and create a more youthful appearance. People who walk slumped over or sit slouched in a chair look old and haggard.

Movement

Movement is also an important part of nonverbal communication. Your gait or how you walk sends a powerful message about you. Have you heard someone described as walking with a "spring in his (or her) step?" That person moves energetically in a way that communicates he or she is happy and confident. A youthful stride will keep you from looking and feeling old.

Often older people walk with a side-to-side movement in their hips and shoulders. This walking pattern, known as Trendelenburg gait, is common in people who need or have recently had a hip replacement. That is why it is so important to attend physical therapy sessions and do exercises at home if you have undergone hip replacement surgery. This abnormal walking pattern will eventually create stress on the knee joints and increase knee problems, often resulting in the need for knee replacement surgery. Because you are in pain, you will be less likely to get the exercise you need, which then impacts so many other body functions.

When gait problems are physical, there are exercises you can do to correct the situation. To test yourself for Trendelenburg, stand in front of a mirror with your hands on your hips. Then lift your right foot off the floor and hold it in that position for as long as you can. Repeat with the left foot. You should be able to hold your foot up for at least 30 seconds per side. If you can't, it would be a good idea to see your doctor, physical therapist, or personal trainer. These trained professionals will be able to give you exercises to improve your gait.

Facial Expression

Facial expressions are fundamental to effective nonverbal communication. Part of being relevant is being approachable. Who would you rather be around—someone with a pleasant facial expression or someone with a neutral expression/frown? Facial expressions create a perception that you are friendly or unfriendly, happy or sad, nice or not nice, in pain or pain free. People react to us based on what they perceive.

Do not underestimate the power of a smile. Smiling not only makes you look happy, it makes you feel happy as well. You can also hear a smile in one's tone of voice. That's why people who work in customer service call centers are instructed to smile when talking to a customer. To reinforce this, often they have a mirror at their workstations so that they can do a self-check throughout their customer interactions.

Eye Contact

In Western civilization, people who maintain good eye contact are perceived as more reliable and honest. Looking someone in the eye conveys respect and interest. One-on-one direct eye contact is becoming more and more difficult as people spend more time with their smartphones and computers. As I will discuss in Chapter 3, "Stay Connected," eye contact is important to building and maintaining relationships.

Mode of Communication Hierarchy

As you reflect on the three elements of interpersonal communication (verbal, visual, and vocal), consider the importance of each communication mode and then choose the one that will result in the most effective communication. The modes of communication in order of the greatest impact and significance are as follows:

- Face-to-face meetings
- Videoconferencing
- Phone calls
- Voice mail
- E-mail

Both face-to-face meetings and videoconferencing incorporate all three elements. Phone calls and voice mail address verbal and vocal. E-mail is last on the list for a reason. It employs only one element (verbal) that people can so easily misinterpret. The receiver, not the sender, will interpret the tone and intent of the message.

Communicating With Different Generations

Many of the people I interviewed stressed the importance of not only socializing with younger folks but really engaging them. Ask them questions to gain insight into their thinking and what is important to them. Find out what apps they are using and websites they are visiting. As the late Stephen Covey, author of *The Seven Habits of Highly Effective People* wrote, "Seek first to understand, then to be understood."

Although I have highlighted specific tips and techniques to enhance communication with each generation, the most effective way to communicate with them is to follow the same best practices you would use in communicating with people regardless of generation.

Regardless of whether you are communicating with millennials, Gen Xers, or your fellow baby boomers, or traditionalists, you must be able to adapt your approach and communication style—particularly with millennials. So, let's start with them. In today's business world, millennials already have a significant presence in the workforce, and they have very specific ideas and opinions about what is relevant or irrelevant. Birtan Collier, profiled in Chapter 8, "Reinvent Yourself," advises "reading about and talking to millennials to learn about what they value and where they're coming from." Casey Johnson, a former attorney with Chubb Insurance, echoes that sentiment: "Getting the input of younger people keeps you young. They inspire me." Following are some tips for communicating successfully with millennials.

Keep It Brief but Meaningful

Whether communicating in written form or orally, get to the point quickly. Keep in mind that millennials have learned to communicate something meaningful in 140 characters or fewer. Although they want information presented concisely, they also want detailed information to help them do their jobs. Thus, provide them with resources so that they can dig deeper and access what they believe they really need.

Use Technology

Millennials are not fans of face-to-face meetings and telephone conversations. They are much more comfortable with and responsive to texts and instant messaging. Many are not fond of e-mails and admit not reading them unless they absolutely must because of work-related expectations. Like many of us, they have adapted to virtual meetings, presentations, and learning situations. Although some don't like the format, they like the freedom and ability to access information any time, any place, and at their convenience. Accept the fact that millennials communicate 24/7, and they expect others to do the same.

What Not to Say

In my research for this book, I interviewed several younger folks and asked them what *older people* do or say that makes them seem old and not relevant. Here are some examples they shared with me:

"I'm having a senior moment."
"Don't get old."
"I'm not as young as I used to be."
"Back in the day…"
"We used to do it…"
"I'm too old for this."
"Getting old is not for sissies."
"I'm technologically challenged."

Don't say things that reinforce in others' minds as well as your own that you are old. More than anything else, don't discuss health issues. Also, avoid talking about the past.

Don't let your language date you. Using words that are clearly outdated and/or noninclusive can be a real turnoff to members of the younger generations. Here are some classic words that need to be eliminated from your vocabulary. If you use words that elicit a snicker or a slight eye roll, stop using them!

Word Usage

Outdated	Contemporary
Dungarees	Jeans
Stewardess	Flight attendant
Videotape	Record
Xerox	Photocopy
Icebox	Freezer
Slacks	Pants
Clicker	Remote

Cash register	Checkout
Mailman	Postal worker
Waiter/waitress	Server
Fireman	Firefighter
Policeman	Police officer
Manpower	Staffing
Oriental	Asian
Salesman	Salesperson
Handicapped	Disabled

Communicating in Writing

Not only do we need to be careful of what we say face to face, but we also need to be mindful of how we come across in writing, especially in e-mails.

Using E-Mail

Love it or hate it, e-mail is a major communication mode, particularly in business. One of the main problems with e-mail (among many) is that we can't see or hear the person sending the message. All we have are the words on the screen. From my experience, many conflicts are caused by e-mail. Two essential elements are missing: visual and vocal. Think about it. Who determines the tone of the e-mail? The receiver, of course. When I am hired to coach people who are engaged in an interpersonal conflict at work, the first thing I tell them is that they can no longer send e-mails to each other. Ideally, they should talk face to face. If that isn't possible due to different locations, then they need to have a conversation on the telephone. I have worked with people in conflict situations who have offices or cubicles next to each other but who communicate only through e-mail.

E-mail is not always the best means of communication. It is difficult to communicate successfully under the best of circumstances. The narrower the communication, the greater the possibility that something will go wrong or be misunderstood as noted earlier. Many e-mail messages should never be sent. They should be handled by a phone call or face to face.

Also, keep in mind that just because you think e-mail is the "best thing since sliced bread," not everyone shares this sentiment. Make it a practice of asking the recipient of your communication, which means he or she would prefer.

When to Use E-Mail

- Use e-mail for presenting information or offering ideas for consideration.
- Use e-mail for a simple exchange of ideas or conversation.
- Use e-mail when other forms of communication are inconvenient.
- Use e-mail to solicit information or ideas from others.
- Use e-mail to document decisions.
- Use e-mail when you need to preserve or archive information.
- Use e-mail to communicate details such as dates, times, numbers, and so forth.

When *Not* to Use E-Mail

In general, e-mail is *not appropriate* for situations that require or rely on interpersonal interaction.

- Don't use e-mail for *official* business.
- Don't send an e-mail message when you are angry or upset. You may live to regret it.
- Don't use e-mail when you are trying to persuade someone to do something.
- Don't reprimand (or even worse, fire) someone via e-mail.
- Don't use e-mail in place of a committee or group meeting when it is important to generate ideas and gain consensus for a decision.
- Don't use e-mail to deal with conflict situations.
- Don't use electronic mail for emergency messages. You have no idea when the message will be read or even if it will be read by the appropriate person.

- Don't use e-mail to conduct personal business. Remember: you are at work, not at home (even if you work from home).

Tips for Using E-Mail

- **_Choose Your Words Carefully._**
  Don't *flame* people, that is, sending a message intended to insult, provoke, or rebuke. Because of the message's brevity and the ease in sending it, people often communicate something they didn't intend. The nuances of oral and interpersonal communication such as tone of voice, silences, eye contact, facial expressions, and so on are difficult to duplicate in writing. We need these signals to help us interpret the meaning beneath the words. Terse messages can be easily misinterpreted by the receiver, who may perceive that you are being sarcastic, critical, or rude. Offended, the receiver *fires off* a nasty response, and the *war of words* begins. The same is true of humor and irony—they can be misinterpreted.
- **_Follow the Rules of Good Writing._**
  E-mail is not an excuse to be sloppy. Keep in mind that you are in a place of business. Although e-mail lends itself to a more informal use of the language, you should still communicate in a business-like manner. In other words, use proper spelling, grammar, and punctuation. Also include a salutation and a closing. Just as with any other form of communication, you project a certain image by the way in which you present yourself.
- **_Avoid "Spam" (Internet Junk Mail)._**
  People's time is precious. They don't have time to read junk mail. Do not send anything unless it is of value to the recipient. That means, avoid sending jokes, chain messages, cartoons, or irrelevant information.
- **_Use Meaningful Subject Lines._**
  The subject line should capture in four or five words what the e-mail message is about.

In other words, the subject line should summarize the most important details of the message. Do not just say, *Hi* or *For Your Information.* Be specific. Because people receive so many e-mails each day, recipients are taking desperate measures to separate the *junk* from the *important stuff.* Many people have started using software filters that automatically screen out e-mail from people or about subjects that the recipient does not want to receive. People, especially those of the younger generations, want to be able to go through their messages quickly and sort out those that are important. A meaningful subject line will help your message stand out and ensure that it gets read.

- **Follow E-Mail Protocol.**
An e-mail does have a language of its own, using letters and characters to add a personal touch or to communicate an emotion. For example, a word typed in all capital letters is the equivalent of shouting and is considered rude. Be aware that many people are inexperienced e-mail users and may not be familiar with the use of abbreviations such as BTW (by the way), TTYL (talk to you later), FWIW (for what it's worth), among others. Inexperienced users may also be baffled by the use of *smilies* (simple strings of characters interspersed in the e-mail text to convey the writer's emotions: :-) represents a smiley face; ;) represents a wink (light sarcasm); :-D means shock or surprise; and :-(is a frown. Emojis have no place in business communication.

- **Remember: E-Mail is Forever.**
E-mail is very public. Even if someone deletes an e-mail message, people can use software programs and online services to access messages on the hard drive. Do not say anything in an e-mail that you would not want someone else to read.

- **Keep It Short.**
E-mail is meant to be brief; therefore, if you have a lengthy document, send it by another means. Keep in mind that the larger the attached document, the longer it takes to download, and the more memory space it fills on the other person's

computer. As a rule of thumb: keep your lines short, keep your paragraphs short, and keep the message short. Remember that the *younger folks* have no patience with long e-mails. They simply won't read them.

- **Answer E-Mail Messages Promptly.**
  Be prompt in responding to action items. Even if you cannot get to it for a while, at least let the sender know you received the message.
- **Eliminate Long Distribution Lists.**
  Send your messages only to the people who need to receive them or who have an active interest in the subject.

Listening: The Forgotten Skill

A much-overlooked element of communication is listening. As we get older, our listening skills seem to get worse. There are several reasons that we are poor listeners. The most obvious is diminished capacity to hear what others are saying, whether it be one-on-one or in a group setting.

If you find yourself answering the wrong question, asking people to repeat what they said, or withdrawing from conversations, please make an appointment right away to have your hearing tested.

In addition to physical issues like hearing loss, another important contributing factor is simply poor listening skills that you may have been practicing your entire life. You may have been able to get away with poor listening habits when you were younger. Now that you are older, poor listening habits may be perceived as hearing loss, and people will respond to you accordingly. Like it or not, poor hearing is often associated with being old. To compensate for hearing loss that is part of the aging process, you must concentrate on practicing good listening skills.

The Importance of Listening

Studies show that we spend 80 percent of our waking hours communicating, and according to research, at least 45 percent of that time is spent listening. Although listening is a primary activity, most individuals are inefficient listeners. Tests have shown that immediately after listening to a

10-minute presentation, the average listener has heard, understood, properly evaluated, and retained approximately half of what was said. And within 48 hours, that drops off another 50 percent to a final 25 percent level of effectiveness. In other words, we comprehend and retain only one-quarter of what we heard.

Why are we such poor listeners? First, we have never really been taught to listen. In school, we are taught speaking, reading, and writing skills, but, in general, there are no courses devoted to listening. Second, most people are so busy talking, thinking about what they are going to say next, or checking their smartphones for e-mails and texts that they miss out on many wonderful opportunities to learn about new things, ideas, and people.

A major component of the listening process is asking open-ended questions and then really listening to the answers. Many years ago, Dale Carnegie in his book, *How to Win Friends and Influence People*, said, "Be a good listener. Encourage others to talk about themselves." By listening, you will discover what motivates your employees to do a good job and your clients to buy your products or services. By listening, you will discover what is really bothering your spouse or children. By listening, you will discover a lot of remarkably interesting people in the world around you—including those from different generations. Listening is the catalyst that fosters mutual understanding and provides us with insight into people's needs and desires so that we can connect with them.

Listening Versus Hearing

Listening is the process of taking in information from the sender or speaker without judging, clarifying what we think we heard, and responding to the speaker in a way that invites the communication to continue. Listening is one of the most important, most underused, and least understood influencing skill. Think about it. How do you feel when someone really listens to you? My guess is that you feel respected and appreciated. When people sense that others are listening to them and trying to understand their viewpoints, people become more open and drop their own barriers. The result is a climate of trust, openness, and mutual respect that leads to greater cooperation.

People confuse hearing with listening. Hearing is the physical part of listening, that is, when your ears sense sound waves. Listening, however, involves interpreting, evaluating, and reacting. Take a moment and complete the following self-assessment to determine your perception of your listening competence and efficiency. Ask yourself the following questions: Do I...

- Maintain eye contact with the speaker in a face-to-face situation?
- Ignore distractions while listening?
- Wait until the speaker is finished before I speak?
- Listen for tone as well as words?
- Try not to over-react to emotionally charged words?
- Listen to understand rather than spend time preparing my next remark?
- Avoid assuming what the other person means by asking questions to ensure understanding?
- Capture the main ideas rather than just the facts when taking notes?
- Refrain from *tuning out* someone I don't like or whose message is boring or contrary to my belief?

How did you do? If you really want to find out if you are an active listener, compare your perception of your listening skills with others' perceptions of you. Ask people close to you such as family members, friends, and co-workers to complete (anonymously, of course) the same assessment by responding to each item with you in mind. You might be surprised by the outcome.

Barriers to Listening

External Barriers

- *Physical environment.* External distractions can be almost anything that involves an outside stimulus. Noise, interruptions, and surroundings can interfere with your ability to listen.

- *Inarticulateness.* A person who is unable to express himself or herself clearly and distinctly creates a tremendous barrier for those listening. If the speaker doesn't speak distinctly, uses words inappropriately, or lacks clarity of thought in expressing ideas, the listener will *tune out.*

Internal Barriers

- *Close-mindedness.* Have you ever tried to talk to someone whose mind was already made-up? Or how about the person who believes that he or she knows the answer? One of the ways you can remain relevant is to approach situations with an open mind and a willingness to do things differently. For example, don't be a dinosaur by saying or thinking, "I'm too old to learn about all this social media."
- *Preoccupation.* Sometimes we just do not pay attention. We may be thinking about something else we need to do or reflecting on something that happened. In either case, the problem is that we are focused on something other than the person and the message at hand. That preoccupation can contribute to the perception that you are not interested or are just not *with it.*
- *Emotional blocks.* We all have emotional reactions triggered by words, topics, or visual stimuli. These triggers can be positive, negative, or neutral. We tend to think that only negative responses interfere with our listening; however, all three can cause us to become poor listeners.

    A negative response, for example, may be elicited when the listener hears a word that makes him or her *see red.* When that happens, the person's emotional response is so intense that he or she *tunes out* anything of value that the speaker may be sharing. We may also become argumentative, creating a major communication breakdown. Neutral responses can also be harmful because they result in apathy or disinterest. Surprisingly, positive emotional responses can interfere with our listening ability as well. Because we like the speaker or are enamored with his

or her topic or viewpoint, we may accept at face value everything he or she is saying. Both negative and positive emotional
triggers are quite evident during political campaigns. In either
case, emotional triggers cause us immediately to evaluate rather
than first comprehending, then interpreting, and finally evaluating properly. One of my emotional blocks is being called
young lady. Clearly, I am over 60 and not young. I find the term
to be condescending.

- *Stereotyping and prejudice.* This barrier refers not only to the
  common prejudices we know such as race, religion, gender,
  age, ethnicity, and so forth, but also prejudices we may have
  about specific individuals. Each of us has personal listening
  biases regarding appearance, manners, and speech. In our
  increasingly diverse society, don't allow your prejudices to get
  in the way.

- *Mind-wandering.* The average person speaks at a rate of
  125 words per minute. Yet an individual can think at a rate
  of 400 to 500 words per minute. As a result, the listener has
  a lot of *leisure* time during which his or her mind wanders,
  thinking about a variety of unrelated topics. Good listeners
  will use this extra time to review, reflect, and summarize the
  message just heard.

- *Defensiveness.* As human beings, we have very definite
  thoughts, opinions, and ideas. When we feel these are being
  questioned or attacked, we become defensive and block
  what the other person is saying. As an example, I find myself
  becoming defensive when someone says, "*You're still working
  at your age?*" or "*You look good for your age,*" or "*When are you
  going to retire?*"

- *Judging.* Some people have already made up their minds that
  the subject is either uninteresting or too difficult. As a result,
  they tune out. Some common responses that indicate the
  listener is judging and not going to be receptive:
  "*I've been there … done that.*"
  "*It's the same old stuff just in a different package.*"

- *Preparing your rebuttal.* Sometimes we are so anxious to *have our say* or express our opinions that we don't listen to the other person's complete message. We are too busy rehearsing in our mind what we are going to say next and trying to find the next opportunity to interject.

Active Listening Benefits

Being an active listener helps you to remain relevant because you are perceived as a person who is actively engaged with whomever or whatever is going on around you. Practicing this often-neglected skill results in many other benefits as well.

- *Keeps communication channels open.* When an atmosphere of trust and openness has been created through active listening, people are more likely to express themselves in a spirit and practice of authentic and ongoing communication.
- *Reduces friction and prevents conflicts.* Poor listening can lead to conflict. We act on what we think we heard, not necessarily on what we did hear. Using active listening skills to clarify and confirm will prevent misunderstandings.
- *Provides opportunities for learning.* When we're talking, we're not learning. Active listening allows us to gather data and information we may not otherwise be exposed to. It's surprising what we can learn just by listening. Alfred Brendel, noted·classical pianist, composer, and poet, noted that "the word 'listen' contains the same letters as the word 'silent'"—just rearranged.
- *Generates ideas.* When people truly listen to one another, they become excited and energized. An environment that encourages people to listen and be listened to is one that ignites both the spirit and the mind and promotes creative thinking.
- *Enlists support of others.* People want and need to feel valued, that what they think and say matters. You are much more likely to support the person who supported you by really listening to what you had to say.

- *Builds and strengthens personal and professional relationships.* Because both people are open and receptive to producing clear communication, they can work together more effectively.
- *Prevents misunderstandings.* As mentioned earlier, we act on what we think we heard, not necessarily what the person meant. If we practice active listening techniques, we ensure that the message sent and received is the same.

Listening Guidelines

Because our listening speed is faster than the other person's speaking speed, there is a lot of *dead* time in the communication process. Often, we fill that void by daydreaming or doing something else like making a *to do* list, doodling, or using our smartphones to check e-mail or text messages. Instead, try using the time to process what the speaker has just said to reach a deeper level of understanding. Following are some guidelines to help you become a better listener.

- *Be aware of your own biases.* It is important that we recognize our own biases regarding subject matter or even our responses to people's backgrounds or appearance. How often have you dismissed comments or ideas from a younger person because they had body piercing, tattoos, or clothing you found offensive or did not like? Simply put, keep an open mind.
- *Identify your emotional triggers.* Certain words or complete messages, ideas, or philosophies can easily arouse our emotions. If you doubt this, just think about your emotional response the next time you hear a politician whose ideology is the opposite of yours. What is your reaction when a younger person challenges your ideas/suggestions or challenges you?
- *Be empathetic and non-judgmental.* Each of us is different with our own quirks and peculiarities. Instead of focusing on distracting behaviors, concentrate on what the speaker is saying. At the end of one of my training sessions with a group of bank branch managers, one of the participants gave me an extremely negative evaluation because he didn't like my eye

makeup. In another situation, a participant complained to the meeting planner because I wore a red suit. In both cases, the participants were not able to concentrate on what I had to say because they were absorbed with what was for them a distraction caused by something in my appearance.

- *Listen to separate fact from opinion.* Avoid jumping to conclusions or making assumptions—warranted or not—about what the other person means. Check it out first.

- *Listen for the feeling of what is being conveyed.* Be aware of nonverbal cues such as gestures, facial expressions, and posture.

- *Take notes.* No matter how good your memory (age considerations aside), you cannot remember everything. Do not, however, attempt to write down every word. In doing so, you are focused on the notetaking process rather than the listening process.

- *Listen for the main idea or thought.* Try to capture in your mind and then put on paper the essence of what the speaker is saying.

- *Give your full attention.* For one-on-one conversations, look the speaker in the eye, lean forward, and encourage the speaker to continue by nodding your head and making verbal comments such as, "That's interesting," or "Tell me more." Even if you find the speaker or the message boring, try to find an area of interest in the speaker's message. Also, as difficult as it may be, do not allow yourself to become distracted by your smartphone, laptop, or other devices.

- *Don't interrupt.* This is a tough one if you have developed that habit. Try to concentrate and inhibit your tendency to interrupt.

- *Limit your own talking.* You cannot talk and listen at the same time. The ancient Greek philosopher Diogenes put it well when he said, "We have two ears and only one tongue in order that we may hear more and speak less."

- *Pay attention to nonverbal cues.* Observe body language. Be patient and sensitive to the other person's feelings and reactions. Several years ago, when I was a bank manager, a vendor dropped into my office and asked if he could talk to me for a few minutes. He spent the next 45 minutes talking at me, telling me all the wonderful things his company could do for me. He never once acknowledged that my body was tensing, my jaw was set, and I was frowning. He was so intent on delivering his message that he ignored the nonverbal cues that I had *tuned him out.*

Active Listening Techniques

Active listening is a two-way process and a shared responsibility. It involves engaging in the following practices:

Clarifying and Confirming

When we listen, we interpret the speaker's message and then respond according to what we think he or she said. Often, our assumptions are incorrect, and our responses can create misunderstandings and even conflict. It is important, therefore, to clarify what we think the speaker has just said by using some of the following approaches:

> "If I understand it, what you're saying is…"
> "What I hear you saying is…"
> "I get the impression that…"

By paraphrasing the content of the message, the speaker can either confirm or further clarify the message, thus ensuring the accuracy of the communication. Clarifying the message is particularly important if you have a hearing loss, if the other person has an accent different from yours, or if you have an emotional reaction to what the person said.

Reflecting Underlying Feelings

Listen between the lines for attitudes, feelings, and motives behind the speaker's words. Be alert to facial expressions, movements, gestures, and tone of voice. Once again, confirm your perceptions by saying the following:

"If that happened to me, I would be upset…"
"I can imagine that you must feel…"
"You sound upset about the situation…"

Inviting Further Contributions

One highly effective way of getting people to be more open and share more about themselves is to ask open-ended questions—those that require more than a *yes* or *no* answer. Open-ended questions start with the words, *who, what, where, when, why,* and *how.* I strongly recommend avoiding *why* questions because they risk coming across as challenging and may cause the other person to become defensive. "Tell me more about…" is also a powerful way to encourage people to expand their comments. Open-ended questions will help you gain valuable insight into the other person's thinking. By asking questions such as "What thoughts have you given to…?" and "How does that fit into…?", you will improve the communication interaction and enhance your effectiveness as an influencer.

Listening is hard work but well worth the effort. Active listening will result in more effective communication and more rewarding relationships.

Communication Checklist

Place a checkmark next to the behaviors you practice on a regular basis.

- I ask for feedback from people whose opinion I value.
- I give feedback that describes the person's behavior and does not judge or attack.
- I practice active listening skills.
- I give the other person my undivided attention when engaged in a conversation.
- I talk about my ideas with energy, excitement, and enthusiasm.

- I show genuine interest in people by encouraging others to talk about themselves.
- I observe and monitor nonverbal cues.
- I adjust my communication style to the situation and the other person.
- I ask open-ended questions to understand the other person's message or position.
- I summarize actions or key points made during a discussion.
- I verify that I understand what is important by paraphrasing what I heard.
- I am clear about the purpose and importance of interactions I initiate.

Take Action!

- Seek out a member of a younger generation (work colleague, friend, grandchild) and discuss what they like to read and watch on television.
- Practice one of the vocal activities described in this chapter.
- Respond to the *Communication Checklist*, and based on your results, choose two practices you would like to improve and then develop a plan to strengthen your skill in those areas.

CHAPTER 3

Stay Connected

Build good relationships and profitable transactions will follow.
—Philip Kotler, American Author

Relationships matter. In today's high-tech world, relationships are becoming increasingly more important. One of the most important takeaways from the pandemic is that people do need people, and they need a feeling of closeness, and closeness has nothing to do with distance. It's about relationships and support systems. During the pandemic, people (especially those who live alone) had to draw on their personal as well as professional connections to overcome a sense of isolation and loneliness.

Personal Relationships

Sometimes people disappoint us, and at times, we disappoint others. Throughout our lives, there comes a time when we must evaluate our relationships and how they impact our lives. Do your friendships lift you up or bring you down? Are you spending precious time and energy hanging on to relationships that seem more like obligations rather than cultivating new ones that energize and support you? Are you around people who drain your energy or who are downright toxic with their negativity and criticism?

Perhaps it is time to apply The KonMari Method to your relationships. The KonMari Method is a unique approach to tidying, developed by Marie Kondo, a Japanese organizing consultant. The central theme of her method is to "keep only those things that speak to the heart and discard items that no longer spark joy. Thank them for their service—then let them go." Although the purpose of this approach relates to tidying your physical environment, perhaps it can apply to your relationships as well.

Reason, Season, or Lifetime

As the poem, "Reason, Season, or Lifetime" (author unknown) states, "People come into our lives for a reason, a season, or a lifetime." Sometimes people come into our lives for a specific purpose or *reason*. It may be to help us through a difficult time or crisis by providing guidance and support and aiding us physically, emotionally, or spiritually. Because the relationship is for a specific purpose, it lasts for a short time, ending when the need no longer exists. For example, when I was diagnosed with breast cancer, two people I hardly knew helped me deal with the emotional trauma.

Most of our relationships are only for a *season*. These seasons are defined by specific periods in our lives such as college or young parenthood. Other seasons may be life-changing events (e.g., disasters), memberships in organizations, or places (e.g. job, neighborhood). When the season ends, generally the relationship ends, too. Sometimes it's difficult to accept that the relationship is over. Don't agonize over it—just let it go and move on. Over my career, I have had the pleasure and privilege of developing personal relationships with some of my long-term client contacts. We would often meet for dinner and began sharing our personal experiences. When the professional relationship ended (even after several years), the personal one gradually faded away.

Lifetime relationships are true friendships and so rare. These are the people who are always there for you in good times and bad. You can tell them anything, and they listen empathetically without judgment. They don't offer advice unless asked, and they tell you things you may not want to hear with love and caring. My lifetime friend, Harriet Rifkin, and I became friends and colleagues when we both worked in banking in Rochester, New York. It could have easily been a *seasonal* relationship because we each left the bank and moved to different cities hundreds of miles apart. But it is truly a lifetime friendship—40 years and counting. Although years may pass between visits and months go by without talking on the phone, when we do connect, it's as though no time has passed. My grandfather used to say, "You can count your true friends on one hand and have fingers left over." He was so right. To me, a friend is someone with whom I can be myself, who brings out the best in me, overlooks the worst in me, and accepts me for who I am—warts and all.

Activity: Reason, Season, Lifetime

To put your relationships in perspective, identify the *reason, season,* and *lifetime* relationships you have had over the years. Write down the categories and then fill them with the names of people who fit in each one, noting what value they brought to your life. As you reflect on the relationships, I'm sure you will conclude that you have indeed been blessed to have known these people.

Professional Relationships

Professional relationships serve specific purposes such as professional development, networking, and business opportunities. No matter where you are in your career or profession, you need to continue to honor existing business relationships and cultivate new ones to remain relevant.

Networking

No matter what profession you are in or where you are on your career path, networking is an essential skill. You may be saying to yourself, "I know how to network. After all, that's how I got where I am today." Although you have been networking your entire career, you can't stop now. You must continue to hone your networking *know-how* to remain relevant and to demonstrate that you are still actively involved in your career/profession. If I had not continued to network, this book would never have become a reality. Every interview I conducted is a result of networking, and the connection to my publisher is tied to a networking event.

Cindy Wollman, a colleague and friend, was scheduled to present at a breakfast networking event for an organization to which we both belong on the topic of her hobby, "Backyard Chickens." I promised to attend to support her. We had the option of participating virtually or in person. I chose virtual. Prior to Cindy's presentation, each in-person attendee delivered a self-introduction. Listening to Vilma Barr's introduction, I was surprised to learn that she is a collections editor for Business Expert Press. I had been searching for a publisher for my book for three years. I immediately contacted her, and the rest is history.

Much to my surprise, over the past few years, I have found that even those who consider themselves to be good networkers are constantly looking for ways to improve their networking skills. Why? Because, like everything else, networking continues to change and evolve. Especially with the introduction of social media, networking has become more involved and sophisticated. However, one thing that has not changed: *networking is about relationships*.

As you reflect on your networking expertise, ask yourself the following questions:

- Are you as effective as you would like to be?
- Do you continue to practice your networking strategies and skills on a regular basis?
- Do you use your network to help other people?
- Do you leverage your connections to build relationships?

If you answered *Yes* to these questions, then you can probably skip this section of the chapter or, better yet, share it with those around you who could use some help in developing their networking skills. However, if you answered *No* to any of them, I encourage you to read on. Keep in mind that this information is meant to be a reminder. Sometimes we tend to take things for granted and rest on our laurels until we are jolted into reality when someone who is younger and more eager has taken our place.

Back to Basics

Networking is making connections and building enduring mutually beneficial relationships. Networking is a supportive system of sharing information and services among individuals and groups. Recognized as the way to get things done in today's environment, networking involves various skills and activities that rely heavily on interpersonal skills and communication. Networking skills help you build a base of influence by developing strong personal and professional relationships. The benefits of networking can be summarized in three simple words: *relationships, opportunities, and resources*. The opportunities very often lead to more business as illustrated and described next.

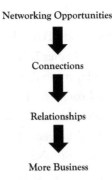

Networking Opportunities

Connections

Relationships

More Business

Figure 3.1 Benefits of networking

Networking Opportunities

Continue to look for opportunities to network. Attend professional networking events through your professional associations and other organizations. Make it a point to attend at least one professional conference a year in your field. In between, attend local meetings and events and join specialty subgroups that often meet in person and keep members connected through various social media platforms.

Make Connections

Take advantage of your networking opportunities to make connections. Do more than exchange business cards and follow up with the usual solicitation e-mail or phone call. Really make connections by meeting for breakfast, lunch, coffee, drinks, and so forth to share information and begin to get to know the people with whom you connected. Find out what they do and what they need. As James Clear writes in his article, "24 Networking Tips That Actually Work," "It's far more important to understand their needs before you tell them about your needs." Focus on listening more and talking less.

Become a Connector

The term *Connector*, was popularized by Malcolm Gladwell in his book *The Tipping Point*. A connector is someone who introduces people who can benefit from each other. Cindy Wollman, a realtor with Berkshire Hathaway Home Services in Glenside, Pennsylvania, mentioned earlier, is a consummate connector. In fact, Chapter 7, "Keep Up With Technology" is a direct result of Cindy connecting me to Paul Dougherty, the techie expert in her office. To be a successful connector like Cindy, you need to have a wide circle of resources such as friends, colleagues, and acquaintances from different backgrounds and varied interests. You also need some personal skills such as active listening to identify potential connections. For example, in a casual lunch conversation, Cindy picked up on my passing remark that I was going to need help with my chapter on technology. When she went back to her office, she talked with Paul to get his permission to connect the two of us. As you will see when you read Chapter 7, he was of tremendous help. This would not have happened if Cindy had not connected us. The message here is simple: get in the habit of making connections for other people. Connecting people is one of the fastest ways to grow your own network. Although this is a simple concept and easy to do, it's rarely practiced. Remember: networking is about helping other people.

Build Relationships

Relationships do not happen overnight. They take time to develop and nurture. Remember: people do business with people they like and trust. The same can be said for referrals. People are not going to refer you to their friends, colleagues, or other business acquaintances if they don't like or trust you.

Nurture your current network of friends and acquaintances by having lunch, connecting via e-mail or telephone, or through social networking media. If you engage in networking opportunities, make connections, and build relationships, you will reap the rewards of increased business. Keep in mind that networking is a process, not an event or series of events. Networking is hard work. It takes time, effort, and patience, but the pay-off is well worth it.

Prepare for a Networking Event

- *Develop a positive mindset.* Prepare yourself mentally and emotionally for the experience. Instead of worrying about what you are going to say and being afraid because you won't know anyone there, tell yourself that this is an exciting opportunity, an adventure. Visualize yourself as confident and in control. Picture what you will wear and see yourself as cool, calm, and collected.

- *Do your homework.* Find out everything you can about who is going to be there: what they do, where they live, what their interests are. If possible, check the list of attendees, identify the people you want to meet, and visit their LinkedIn profiles before you go.
- *Define your purpose.* Be clear about what you want to get from the experience. Do you want to establish contacts, gain business leads, or gather information?
- *Prepare your own introduction.* In preparation for your networking events, make sure you have a good elevator speech/pitch (also called your 60-second *commercial* or self-sell) that is clear, concise, relevant, and makes people say, "Tell me more."
- *Prepare two or three topic questions.* You might ask people what drew them to this organization or event. You could also inquire about how far they had to travel to get there, or how long they have been involved with the organization.

The Art of Conversation

The first place to start in developing your networking strategy is to fine-tune your conversation skills. Being known as a good conversationalist can enhance your image and create or reinforce a person's impact on others. Three words will help you shine as a conversationalist: *listen, learn, link.* To master the art of conversation, your primary goal is to actively listen to learn as much as you can about the other person and establish a common link.

Here are some basics to help you shine in any situation:

Introduce yourself. Be assertive. Don't be afraid to walk up to a group of people or an individual and introduce yourself. If you start with a small cluster of people, move close to the group but remain on the outer perimeter. If no one notices you and asks you to join in, listen attentively to the conversation, then at an appropriate moment make a relevant comment and then give your brief introduction. Don't be discouraged if people don't welcome you with open arms. Sometimes it takes several tries to find a *fit*.

One of the big mistakes I see demonstrated by seasoned professionals is that they tend to gravitate toward each other. Instead of trying to connect with someone new, they cluster together during the networking event, resulting in missed opportunities to begin a new relationship. When I attend a networking event where there are people I know, I say my brief *hellos* and then seek out those whom I do not know and introduce myself. In particular, I look for people who are standing by themselves—sometimes literally in a corner. They are uncomfortable, maybe even scared, and would be relieved if someone approached them with a warm smile and made them feel welcomed. Because you made that person feel comfortable, you may have made a friend for life.

Start or stimulate a conversation. Begin by asking open-ended questions to get people talking. Here are some possible openings you might try: "What do you think about...?" "How did you happen to...?" "What brought you to this event?" "Tell me more about...?" The important thing is to get the other person to talk about himself or herself, but be careful that you don't sound like an interrogator.

Business attorney William Maston stresses the importance of "being in the moment with someone" and really engaging with them. One of the ways he does this is by asking questions. As Bill puts it, "Ask great questions and listen. Inquisitiveness is a source of inspiration." He further asserts that "people want to be challenged by questions," and by engaging people through questions, you can "overcome age barriers and create a positive perception."

Listen actively. *Listen* is the first part of my three-part formula in the art of conversation. Active listening begins with a genuine interest in the other person and what he or she has to say. We listen actively and attentively to *learn* something about the individual. For a review of active listening tips, you may want to revisit Chapter 2, "Communicate Clearly." Remember that the greatest compliment you can pay a person is to listen without interrupting or cutting the person short.

Look for commonalities. This is the linking part. Once you have asked open-ended questions and engaged in actively listening to identify common interests, the next step is to comment and *link* to a similar situation or idea. I cannot begin to tell you how many times asking those open-ended questions has opened the door to opportunities and connections. Those questions have led to discovering commonalities such as knowing the same people, living in the same town, graduating from the same university, working for the same company (or industry), and so forth. You get the picture.

Avoid "I-Itis." One of the biggest mistakes people make during conversations is that they spend much of the time focusing on themselves, expounding on what they do or think. Good conversationalists watch their listeners for cues when they may have begun to bore others.

Choose appropriate topics. Good conversationalists are also well-read and well-informed and can talk with anyone on a variety of subjects. They know when it is appropriate to talk about particular topics and include everyone in the group by bringing up topics of general interest, not limited to any specific gender, age, or background. A good conversationalist is sensitive to others and chooses topics and words that do not offend.

Part of remaining relevant is to sound relevant. Make sure people know you have outside interests, particularly those that you have in common with the people with whom you are engaged in conversation. Let people know (subtly, of course) that you work out, play golf, do yoga, go hiking, and so forth. It should go without saying that topics to avoid include ethnic or off-color jokes, sexist remarks, surgery, health issues, dieting, catastrophes, death, religion, or politics.

Building Relationships

Remember: networking is about helping other people. It's also about building relationships. Start out by focusing on being friendly and helpful. Find out about what they're working on or what they're interested in. If you have a resource that is related (article, book, and information), send it to them after meeting them and periodically thereafter.

Never underestimate the importance of including in your network people from diverse backgrounds and particularly those from different age groups. Much has been said and written about age gaps and the problems they create in the workplace. You will find that age differences disappear or at least are minimized when we build relationships.

> *Become friends with people who aren't your age. Hang out with people whose first language isn't the same as yours. Get to know someone who doesn't come from your social class. This is how you see the world. This is how your grow.*
>
> —Roumaissa

Using LinkedIn As a Networking Tool

I imagine that many of you reading this book have a LinkedIn account. However, how many of you are really using it as a key networking tool? I must confess that I fall short in this area myself; however, it's high on my *To Do* list for this year. LinkedIn is the world's largest professional networking platform, and, therefore, the most influential. Those of us who use it only to keep in touch with colleagues, clients, and co-workers are missing many opportunities to really connect and build relationships with others. Here are some tips for using LinkedIn to establish a presence and help you remain relevant.

Complete Your Profile

I am amazed at how many people have not made the effort to create a robust profile. Your profile is your opportunity to showcase who you are, what you do, and your professional accomplishments. It also provides insight into how you can benefit the potential client who is looking for someone to help solve a business problem or perhaps even collaborate on a project.

Go to your LinkedIn account and follow the instructions for completing your profile. Make sure you have a recent professional photo, a summary of what you do and what you offer, as well as a description or examples of your work. Keep in mind that the more complete your profile, the greater the likelihood that people who are *searching* will be directed to you.

Leverage "My Network"

The My Network feature enables you to connect with other LinkedIn users by inviting people to connect and accepting invitations to connect. Regarding accepting invitations, there are mixed opinions. Some people believe in accepting all invitations; others will accept invitations from those they know (or want to know). As mentioned earlier, networking involves connecting two people to one another. My Network enables you to make those connections.

In addition to your primary or first-degree connections, you will also have *second-degree* connections created through your *first-degree* connections. Note that the more *first-degree* connections you have, the more likely you are to *pop up* on the LinkedIn search engine.

Give and Receive Recommendations and Endorsements

Personal testimonials are effective ways to highlight your skills and expertise. In this section, you can post recommendations and endorsements from your professional connections. These are particularly important for those of us who deliver professional services. So, how do you get these endorsements and recommendations? You ask for them! By the same token, offer to write testimonials for others.

Chapter 7, "Keep Up With Technology" addresses more ways LinkedIn can help you remain relevant.

Networking Checklist for Seasoned Professionals

Check your networking savvy by asking yourself the following questions. Do I...

- Always carry business cards and practice business card etiquette?
- Attend a professional networking event every month?
- Have a 30-second self-introduction that I can use in any situation?
- Use LinkedIn to comment/congratulate people on their work anniversaries, new positions, promotions, and accomplishments?

- Have breakfast, lunch, dinner, drinks, or coffee with colleagues at least every two months?
- Talk to and/or sit with people I don't know at a business-related event?
- Ask open-ended questions to find out more about the person to whom I'm talking?
- Make a concerted effort to involve others in conversations?
- Follow up with a handwritten note, telephone call, or e-mail after I meet someone new?
- Thank people via e-mail, handwritten note, or telephone call when they have helped me?
- Ask people what I can do to help them?
- Contact current and former clients just to *check in* every few months?
- Approach an individual or small group of strangers at a social or business function and introduce myself?
- Send articles to colleagues, clients, business associates that I think they would find helpful or informative?
- Introduce people to each other who I believe would mutually benefit from the connection?

Mentoring

By now in your career, I am sure you are familiar with mentoring. Perhaps you have had the benefit of having one or more mentors over the past decades. Very likely, you have already served as a mentor to others. From your vast experience as a mentor and mentee, you probably know and can cite the benefits of mentoring, especially from the mentee's position. What I am proposing here is that you think about the benefits of being a mentor and how being a mentor can help you remain relevant.

Be a Mentor

One of the ways you can benefit from being a mentor is collaborative learning. As you help others improve their skills, you will improve yours as well. You will find that you can learn a lot from your mentee such as new strategies and ways of doing things as well as different ideas and perspectives, Furthermore, because your mentee is closer to the action, that is, functioning *in the trenches*, you can learn a lot about what is going on at the ground level and use that insight to help you propose new and better ways of operating the business.

Working with a mentee requires you to be on your toes and ready to respond to challenging questions your mentee is likely to pose. Furthermore, your willingness to help people at a more junior level will send a signal that you are approachable and not some stodgy *over-the-hill* person just waiting to retire. *One caveat: be sure you are up to date on what the younger folks want and need as they are building their careers and be careful of how you interact with them.* Don't come across as a parent or someone who is out of touch with what is going in today's world. Remember: they don't care about "the good old days," or "the way we used to do it."

Being a successful, *with it* mentor will help in developing relationships that will not only last a lifetime but will continue to benefit you as the mentee moves along in his or her career. Your mentee will remember how helpful you were and may have opportunities to bring you along when they make a move to a higher position or a new company. They will keep you in mind when they need a speaker for a professional organization to which they belong or hire you for a consulting assignment.

Get a Mentor

Reverse mentoring is not new. Jack Welch, former CEO of General Electric, implemented it in 1999. However, it did not really *catch on* until technology became more mainstream. Simply put, reverse mentoring is when older managers and executives are paired with younger employees who teach the seasoned folks about modern technology, including social media. Whether you are employed in a large corporation, own a small business, or are a sole practitioner, there is no doubt that staying on top of technology trends and best practices are important skills for *those of a certain age* to have at least a working knowledge and understand how they can use technology, especially social media, to remain relevant.

I have experienced the benefits of mentoring firsthand. Many years ago, when I was a bank training director in Rochester, New York, I managed and served as a mentor to a group of management trainees. About a year after I started the management training program, I left the bank to start my own consulting business and gradually lost contact with my trainees. Five years after starting my own business, my husband was promoted and transferred to the Philadelphia area, where I had to start my business all over again. As part of my networking efforts in a new area, I had been asked to speak at a New Jersey chapter of the American Society for Training and Development. Much to my surprise and delight, Kim McConnell, one of my former trainees was in the audience. We reconnected, and she told me she had become a bank trainer largely because of me and had relocated to New Jersey to take a job with one of the bank's subsidiaries. Shortly thereafter, she left the bank and took a training position with another company. She continued to progress in training responsibilities in other companies. All in all, she brought me in as a training consultant for three companies. When she left her last corporate position to start her own business, we continued to collaborate and work on projects together. That relationship has lasted nearly 40 years.

Many larger organizations have structured reverse-mentoring programs, just as they probably have traditional mentor–mentee programs. For example, AXA, a global leader in insurance and asset manager, has a formal program that involves six one-hour sessions, during which the younger employee works with the older employee to help him or her learn the basics of the latest and most popular technologies. They show them how to perform various tasks using their smartphones, tablets, or laptops.

If you do not have the advantage of access to a formal reverse mentoring program, do not let that deter you. Seek out your own mentor from any department within your organization. In addition to learning how to use social media for business purposes, you can learn about other technology-related issues such as privacy and data protection. Not only will you gain confidence related to using technology, but your ability also to understand and use technology will go a long way to help you remain relevant in the eyes of your colleagues and team members.

As with traditional mentoring, you will build relationships with your *techno-savvy* mentor. As mentioned earlier, that can pay off in ways that you might not even begin to imagine. You create a mutually beneficial or symbiotic relationship by learning from each other. You learn how to use technology and the younger person gains valuable insight into what it takes to become a successful professional.

Not only do mentoring programs and activities benefit the individuals involved, they also go a long way to close the generation gap. The more people interact with each other, the more they get to know each other, and they begin to see each other as people. Perceptions will change. The younger folks will no longer see you as "that old person who is past his or her prime" but someone from whom they can learn. The more experienced person will come to see "those kids who think they know everything and feel entitled" as great learning resources as well.

Volunteer

I am sure that at this point in your life, you have had many volunteer experiences and probably continue to do so. Volunteer experiences are great ways to build relationships, and the opportunities are limitless. Through volunteer experiences, you meet and interact with people whose backgrounds may be quite different from yours. As a volunteer, I would imagine you have reaped the benefits of personal satisfaction that comes from helping others. But let's look at how volunteer experiences can help you remain relevant.

Internal Volunteering

Perhaps you have been with an organization for a number of years and have had many experiences chairing or serving on committees. In fact, those experiences and the exposure you received probably helped you get where you are today. You may be tempted to say to yourself, "I've been there, done that" or "They [the powers that be] know my track record."

Don't rest on your laurels. People easily and quickly forget what you did in the past. I have also heard seasoned professionals say, "It's time to let the younger folks take over. I paid my dues." If that is how you really feel, that's fine. However, *if you want to remain relevant, this is not the time to sit back and let the younger folks push you aside.* Continue to volunteer to chair business-focused committees and organization-sponsored events. Better yet, come up with your own new initiatives and pitch them to the appropriate people. Show those around you that you are still a vital contributor.

External Volunteering

In my circle of colleagues, friends, and acquaintances, I know a lot of people who volunteer. Similarly, I know a lot of people who do not. The biggest excuse I hear from those folks is, "I don't have enough time." The paradox is that the people who are the busiest in their professional lives are also those who make the time to volunteer.

I have volunteered almost my whole life. As a child and teenager, I volunteered through the Girl Scouts, 4-H, and church. As a young adult, I became more involved in community activities such as the Jaycees. Once I entered the business world, my volunteer activities centered around professional organizations and social clubs. Most recently, I have decided to take my own advice and volunteer (and now serve on the board) at Providence Animal Center (PAC), a no-kill animal rescue organization in Media, Pennsylvania.

Through my experiences and interactions with volunteers and staff members, I have learned (and continue to learn) so much about animal welfare. I have also had the joy and benefit of meeting and working with people of different ages and backgrounds. This personally enriching experience has expanded my network of personal and professional relationships. As an aside, the opportunity to become involved with PAC is linked to networking and relationships with people in a social organization to which I belong.

We all know that volunteering helps others, improves our communities, and strengthens your social network. Knowing that we have made a difference in the lives of others makes us feel good and feeling good enhances our psychological and emotional well-being. (More about that in Chapter 6, "Seek Harmony.") What you may not have thought about is how volunteering can help you remain relevant. Let's look at those benefits.

Benefits of Volunteering

Meet New People and Build Relationships

Throughout this chapter, I have discussed the importance of building relationships as an aid to remaining relevant. Interacting with people who come from diverse backgrounds but who share a common interest is rewarding in and of itself. People build closer relationships, make better connections, and experience greater satisfaction through these shared experiences. The overwhelming majority of people I interviewed stressed the importance of interacting with and building relationships with people of all ages and backgrounds. In particular, they emphasized the benefits of surrounding yourself with people who are younger. As Bill Maston asserts, "A natural tendency in aging is letting your world get smaller. Never isolate yourself with respect to age."

Improve Mental and Physical Health

As a result of increased socializing, people experience better brain function and lower risk for depression and anxiety. It reduces stress and improves our overall health and well-being. According to a report from the Corporation for National and Community Service, research demonstrates that volunteering leads to better health. Those who volunteer "have lower mortality rates, greater functional ability, and lower rates of depression later in life than those who do not volunteer." Research conducted by the Harvard School of Public Health shows that "people who volunteered spent fewer nights in the hospital" than non-volunteers. Other studies noted that volunteers had better health, more stamina, and lower stress levels. When we feel good mentally and physically, we perform better on the job. *Performing better on the job demonstrates that we are indeed relevant.*

Maintain Visibility

No matter where you are in life or your career, visibility is important but even more so as you age. If you don't remain visible, people may forget about you and conclude that you have lost interest in your work, have health issues, or are just coasting until retirement. According to Thomas J. Lynch, Vice President and Portfolio Manager for The Haverford Trust Company in Radnor, Pennsylvania, "One of the best ways to remain relevant is to maintain visibility both socially and businesswise. That includes being active in organizations, especially in leadership roles." Paul Heintz, an attorney with Obermayer Rebmann Maxwell & Hippel, reflects that sentiment by remaining active in the Philadelphia Bar Association and serving as a guest lecturer for organizations on the topics of cybersecurity as well as ethics and technology, two very relevant topics.

Develop New Skills and/or Expertise
As you volunteer your time and talents, not only will you continue to hone your existing skills, but you may also develop new knowledge and skills, particularly if you volunteer in a new industry. This can be particularly helpful if you decide to switch fields or start your own consulting business—more about this in Chapter 8, "Reinvent Yourself."

So, here is the bottom line: If you already volunteer, continue to do so. In fact, you may even want to add another cause to your volunteer list. If you don't volunteer, start now!

Take Action!

- Choose two items from the *Networking Checklist for Seasoned Professionals* and act on them.
- Seek out a volunteer opportunity in your community.
- Make a list of clients and colleagues with whom you have not connected in a while. Contact one person a week and arrange to get together or chat on the phone.

CHAPTER 4

Update Your Image

Perception is real even when it is not reality.
—Edward de Bono, Physician, Psychologist, Author, Inventor

We hear and read a lot every day about image. Politicians, corporations, movie stars, even countries are concerned about image. Image is also important in our daily lives—both personally and professionally. Image is the *perception* others have of us. How others perceive us is determined by several factors including our appearance, the way we communicate, and what we do and say.

People form an impression of you within the first few seconds. That impression helps them make decisions about you, your competence, credibility, and so forth. Appearance includes your physical presence such as how you dress, your body language, and grooming. We have all heard that "you can't judge a book by its cover." But many people do. If you ever doubt this, observe how differently you are treated when you are dressed up versus when you are wearing jeans and a sweatshirt. Never underestimate the power of perception.

You may be thinking, "Why do I need to worry about what I look like? Here I am in my 60s (70s or even 80s), and I dress and act the part of a highly successful person. I have nice, maybe even expensive clothes, shoes, and accessories. My 'look' helped me get to where I am today. I've made it." Not so fast.

Packaging is important. That's why companies change the look of their products frequently. We need to do the same. Many of the dos and don'ts we were concerned about when we started our careers such as what we wear, how we look, what we say have changed. That well-made suit or dress may make mark you as *old*. The good news is that you can update it with accessories or with the help of a good tailor. As we modify or change our packaging, the new image must still be congruent with your style preference, lifestyle, type of business you are in, budget, and body type.

Perception

To me, age is just a number; it is not who I am. Other people in my age group feel the same. During our interview, interior designer Rosa Cucchia said, "I really don't think about how old I am. I think you get old when you stop doing what you love to do." Another example of this mindset is skydiver Paul Moorehead who is still doing solo jumps at age 90 and asserts that "90 is the new 60." Sometimes we must realize that not everyone sees it that way. I had another *aha* moment when we were on vacation at one of the Delaware beaches.

While we were waiting to be seated for dinner at a local restaurant, we decided to order a drink at the bar and stood next to a couple probably in their late 40s or early 50s. This is the interaction between the couple and us:

Wife (to me): How old are you?
Me: Oh, my. I can't believe you asked.
Wife: My husband and I have a bet. My mother is 76, and I think you look younger.
Me: I am.
Husband (obviously embarrassed): Let me pay for your drinks.
My Husband: No, thanks. We already paid.
Husband (handing me a $20 bill) Well, then, this is for the next round.

Self-Assessment: How I Want to Be Perceived

You may find it helpful and enlightening to start this section with a self-assessment by asking yourself the following questions:

- What words would you use to describe your physical appearance/presentation?

- What words do you think others would use to describe your physical appearance/presentation? (You may want to ask a trusted friend to help you with this.)
- Are the two lists congruent?
- What, if anything, would you like to change?

Just for Women

Appearance

The first place to start in addressing your appearance is with what you wear. A youthful appearance can add years to your career and dollars to your income. To create and maintain a youthful appearance, you need to look pulled together with the appropriate clothing along with attractive shoes, handbag, jewelry, and hairstyle. Observe what the younger women are wearing, but don't try to look like you are in your 20s or 30s. You want to maintain a youthful appearance by wearing clothes that are not outdated or old looking.

Purge and Purchase

If you have been wearing the same business attire for more than 10 years, it's time to overhaul your wardrobe. That doesn't mean you have to get rid of everything and start over. It does mean you will need to do some purging and replacement, keeping in mind that what looked good on you in the 60s, 70s, and 80s will make you look dated now that you are in your 60s, 70s, and 80s. Women, don't dress like your daughter or granddaughter, but don't dress like your mother either. Men, if you are still wearing the *Bill Cosby-style* sweaters from the 1980s, it's time to get rid of them.

Ladies, do you ever look in your closet for something to wear, begin trying on one outfit after another, and conclude nothing looks good on you? Even though you may weigh the same as you did when you wore certain clothes a year ago, now they just don't look right. How did that happen? Well, our bodies shift, and women are particularly prone to putting on inches around the mid-section, causing us to look and feel frumpy or matronly. Everything changes as we age—hair, skin tone, body composition. Even if your weight has remained the same for the past 30 years, it's a safe bet that gravity and the aging process have changed your body composition.

To go from *frumpy* to *fabulous*, engage the services of an image consultant or a personal shopper from one of the major department stores in your area. Personal shoppers will help you build on what you have and get rid of those items you haven't worn in five years or more. They will show you how to update your wardrobe with scarves, jewelry, shoes, and handbags. As a rule, stick with classic pieces and update with carefully selected accessories. You may need to take your clothes to a seamstress or tailor who can make the necessary alterations so your clothes fit your body well. Image consultants can also help you identify the styles and colors that look good on you.

You may remember the *color wheel* from the 1970s that helped people identify what colors looked good on them by season. If you are an *autumn* person, your colors are earth tones (brown, orange, yellow, and so forth); a *winter* person looks good in jewel tones such as teal, emerald green, royal blue, purple; *spring* people should wear pastels (light pink, blue, lilac, yellow); and *summer* people can wear any color that has a blue undertone as well as soft pinks and sea green.

Today, it's much simpler. People's color preferences are labeled as *warm, cool,* or *neutral.* Color theory is fascinating, and I encourage you to define your color palette by seeking the help of a professional color expert. You can also start by simply doing an Internet search on color wheels or palettes, and there are many sites that will help you identify what colors look good on you. Also, take note of the compliments you receive about your clothing, particularly when someone says, "That color looks great on you."

According to Carol Davidson, image consultant and founder of Styleworks in New York City, the best colors for women over 50 are the following:

- Periwinkle
- Medium violet
- Watermelon red
- Warm pink

- Teal
- Medium turquoise
- Medium gray
- Soft white

Black is considered too severe for older women. If, however, you just cannot bear to give up your black outfits, you can brighten the look with scarves and other accessories. Also, be open-minded and embrace navy, charcoal, and taupe as alternatives to black.

Shoes

Let's talk shoes—one of my favorite subjects. Shoes can make or break an outfit. Unfortunately, as we age, our feet change as well. They get longer and wider. At this point in our lives, many of us have foot *issues*, caused by years of wear and tear from poorly fitting shoes or high heels. Women, if teetering around on four-inch heels is no longer your *cup of tea*, you can still look stylish (and be comfortable) by choosing a lower heel, kitten heel, wedge, or a cute trendy flat.

Briefcase or Handbag

A briefcase or handbag is an investment, and it says a lot about you, so buy the best you can afford. Trendy tote bags are a great alternative to briefcases for women. Should you choose to go that route, make sure it is a quality product. Observe what younger professional women are carrying to hold all their *stuff.*

Eyewear

As we age, our vision changes, and we may need to wear bifocals. One sure way of making yourself look dated is to wear reading glasses on the tip of your nose. Make an investment in good-looking trendy eyewear with a built-in reader. Consider contact lenses or Lasik surgery. Whatever you decide to do, consult a reputable eye care professional.

Hair

For both men and women, choose a hair color and style that flatters you and is up to date. This may sound sexist, but men with gray hair look distinguished and are regarded as sources of knowledge and experience, but a woman with gray hair is viewed as just old. Stay away from very dark hair color. Remember, skin tone changes. Nothing looks more ridiculous than a color that looks like it came from a bottle of black shoe polish. Find a good colorist who can help you choose the right color for your age and skin type. Also find a good hair stylist who can cut and style your hair that is not only contemporary but also complements the shape of your face.

If you decide to color your hair for a younger, more *with it* look, consider adding some highlights. If you opt for a solid darker color, consider that the nice shiny dark brown hair you had in your 40s will probably look very harsh on you now that you are older. Keep in mind that as we age our pigmentation softens, and we appear to lose color. If you don't want to give up your dark hair, opt for a softened version of the color. If you have thinning hair, a short cut will add volume. For those with fine limp hair, in addition to a shorter haircut, choose hair products such as volumizing shampoo and setting gel. Hair extensions are also a way to combat thinning hair.

Nails

Nail polish and shape are very personal, so it is difficult to really address what you should or should not do. As with women of any age, the important thing is to make sure your nails are manicured. As a rule of thumb, keep your nails short and in a squarish oval shape. Filing your nails in long points will make you look dated. As to nail color, there are so many choices! Keep in mind that as you get older, your skin becomes thinner and thus is more likely to show your bluish veins. If that is the case, then you should avoid cool colors such as blues and greens and blue-based reds and plums. Nude nail polish is always an excellent choice. It has anti-aging power and goes with everything. If you have brown spots on your hands due to too much sun exposure, stay away from deep and dark browns, blacks, or purples. Instead, choose cranberry, burnt creamy plums, or blood reds. Light and soft shades of pink are also good choices. One color to avoid is yellow because it tends to emphasize the dryness and details of your hands.

Makeup

Makeup is also very personal and individualized. One thing is certain. If you are still using same makeup techniques you applied 10 years ago, then it's time for a change. To begin, you need to tend to the condition of your skin with proper cleansing, exfoliating, and nourishing your skin. Make sure to eat lots of vegetables and drink plenty of water. It should go without saying that you need to stay out of the sun. Because older faces are colorless, choose a makeup base that evens out the irregularities in skin tone, then add a pink-toned blusher and a lipstick that complements your skin tone. Be sure to use face, eye, and lip primers to keep your makeup in place for hours.

Older faces are heavier at the bottom than younger ones. To combat this problem, use a highlighter on the top of your cheekbones and on the brow bones to brighten your face and make your eye makeup look better. Eye makeup is tricky—especially as we age. Harsh, overdone eyes will make you look dated. In choosing eye makeup, keep in mind that dark colors make things recede, while light colors bring everything forward. If you need help, seek out the services of a makeup professional and not the sales associate at your department store's cosmetic counters.

Eyebrows

As we age, women's eyebrows tend to become sparse, and many women tend to compensate by drawing eyebrows with an eyebrow pencil, a technique that looks artificial as well as dated. To prevent looking like a painted doll's face, there are three ways to get full, groomed brows. One way, of course, is what we have been doing for years: tweezing stray hairs underneath and/or at the tail and then filling in with a pencil or colored gel wand. The second technique is to apply a brow serum daily to grow hairs and strengthen them. A third way is to dye them. This would involve an in-salon treatment where dye is applied to the hairs. A variation of that (and more expensive) is microblading, a procedure that involves a technician who uses a super-skinny blade to imbed semi-permanent pigment in your eyebrows. You could also try tattooing your eyebrows.

Teeth

Our teeth have taken a *beating* over the years, and they are such an important part of our appearance. Of course, it is understood that you need to see a dentist regularly for a checkup and cleaning, but if you find yourself self-conscious about the look of your teeth, consider cosmetic dentistry. A smile is so important in communicating confidence and approachability. You may need to invest in whitening or straightening depending on your financial resources. Also, for some, dental implants may be in order.

Just for Men

Wardrobe

Business attire for both men and women is becoming increasingly more confusing, especially for men. Traditionally men had few choices in work-related clothing. The official *uniform* was (and still is in many places) the suit, dress shirt, and tie. Times are changing primarily due to the influence of younger workers in the workplace and working from home. From law firms to investment banks, professional attire is becoming much more casual. Even conservative Wall Street has accepted and adjusted to a more flexible dress code, ditching the suit and tie in most professional settings. What you wear to work is influenced not only by employees' preferences but also by the employer's location (city or region) and by the organization's culture and type of business.

As a rule of thumb, observe what younger people (particularly those in power positions) wear and then follow their example. If you are the only person in the office wearing a tie, you are going to look outdated, and people will regard you as such. However, even if you are in a more casual work environment, there are still some basic guidelines you should follow when selecting your clothing and accessories, regardless of culture or climate.

According to Brian Lipstein, president and CEO of Henry A. Davidsen, specialists in high-end, custom-tailored clothing and image consulting for professional men, located in Philadelphia, "Your wardrobe is a huge component of what makes a first impression. It's your image. In the business world, that image can make the difference between gaining the competitive edge or yielding to the competition."

Lipstein has created the "3 Pillars of Style" to provide a roadmap any man can follow to ensure that he's dressed in a permanently stylish way that is still unique to him.

- The first pillar addresses fit. The best way to ensure a good fit is to have clothes made for you. However, if this approach is beyond your budget, make sure you take your off-the-rack purchase to a good tailor.
- The second pillar is color coordination. Some people seem to have a *natural eye* for coordinating colors. If that is not one of your areas of strength, do a Google search on *color wheel* and use that to help you identify what colors go together.
- Pattern coordination, the third pillar, deals with pattern coordination. When coordinating different patterns such as stripes, dots, checks, and paisleys, scale is important. For example, you would match large-scale patterns to small-scale patterns. For more information on the three pillars, visit the Henry A. Davidsen website (https://henrydavidsen.com) and search for the January 8, 2019 blog, "The 3 Pillars of Style."

While men's clothing is less complicated than women's, there are certain guidelines men should be aware of and adhere to if they want to look stylish and not dated. Let's start with suits and sport coats. Look in your closet and determine how long those garments have been there. Keep in mind that as we age, our body shape changes, and we are likely to become shorter as well. So, to maintain proper fit, seek the services of a good tailor. The length of a coat is very important. A longer coat will make a man look top heavy and thus shorter. Shortening the coat is not a good idea. In fact, a reputable tailor will advise against it. So, make an investment in quality suits and sport coats and consult with a professional image consultant.

One wardrobe staple that every professional man should have is the navy blazer. Depending on what type of shirt you wear with it, the blazer can be casual or somewhat dressy. Speaking of shirts, dress shirts should fit. Often, men pay less attention to the fit of their shirts because (a) they don't think anyone will notice because the shirt is under a jacket/coat, (b) they are unaware of how a shirt should fit, or (c) they don't want to spend the money to buy custom-made shirts or have them adjusted by a tailor. Rest assured that people will notice. An ill-fitted dress shirt is uncomfortable, ruins your image, and communicates that you don't care how you look. Off-the-rack shirts rarely fit as they should. That is why you need to spend the money to make sure your shirts fit your entire body. Believe it or not, there are seven elements of fit:

1. Collar fit
2. Shoulder fit
3. Torso fit
4. Sleeve fit
5. Sleeve cuff
6. Sleeve length
7. Bottom hem length

If you choose to buy premade shirts, the fit considerations noted are still the same. To ensure you are purchasing a high-quality shirt, seek the advice of sales associates in upscale menswear shops and department stores. In addition to the elements of fit, pay attention to a few basic do's and don'ts. For example, if you wear a button-down shirt, don't wear a tie. Also, don't wear a shirt with pockets. The collar spread is important. If you are on the heavy side, your collar spread should be wider to balance your face.

Ties and Handkerchiefs

Choosing ties can be tricky because there are so many options. You must take into consideration the style and color of the shirt as well as the color and style of the suit or sport coat. In general, a subtle patterned tie is always appropriate for older men, and it will pull your look together. Once again, I recommend an image consultant or a salesperson experienced in men's clothing to help you choose the right tie. The trend in tie width changes frequently. Trending now (as of this writing), your tie's width should be 3–3.5 inches. In addition, ties should balance your body.

What about pocket squares (also known as pocket handkerchiefs or suit handkerchiefs)? According to menswear fashionistas, a pocket square is a must. If you are wearing a blazer, sport coat, or suit, you must include a pocket square to have a pulled-together look. There are several ways to fold a pocket square (straight fold, two points, three points, nonchalant). The type of fold depends on what type of jacket you are wearing as well as the occasion. Whatever you do, don't use a pre-folded pocket square or one that matches your tie. The pocket square should complement the tie in terms of color and pattern.

While we are about handkerchiefs, never ever use a handkerchief instead of a tissue to blow your nose. Quite frankly, other people, especially the younger set, find that disgusting!

Footwear—Shoes and Socks

Just as with women, your shoes need to be appropriate for the occasion and what you are wearing. After all, you wouldn't (shouldn't) wear sneakers with a suit. Men are much more limited in their shoe selections, but following some basic guidelines will ensure that you will look put together. A cap-toe Oxford is very versatile. It's dressy but still contemporary. In general, brown or tan shoes are more casual, while black shoes are more formal. Also, make sure your shoes and belt match.

It goes without saying that your socks should match and have no holes or visible stains. Choose excellent quality socks that match your trousers and make sure that they are long enough that when you cross your legs, there is no bare skin exposed. Your socks should also match the dress level of the rest of your ensemble (e.g., black tie versus casual).

Hair

We addressed the issue of color and cut earlier under the section for women. For men with thinning hair, keep your hair short. Image consultants suggest that if you are losing your hair, any style that is more than ½ inch long is a no-no. On the other hand, if you are lucky enough to still have a nice crop of hair, don't ruin your image by wearing it too long.

But what about baldness? Some men are quite happy and comfortable with their baldness and take pride in their shaved heads. Other men, particularly with thinning hair, are very self-conscious and want to increase hair volume. There are several options available such as medication, hair plugs, or hair pieces. Your choice will depend on a variety of factors, including personal preference and cost.

What about facial hair? Beards and mustaches tend to go in and out of style. A great website for men's grooming products as well as tips and techniques for caring for your beard is The Grooming Lounge (www.groominglounge.com). They also have a guide for choosing a beard shape for your face. Check out their video that addresses *beard lines*. Beard lines are the "guiding lines that help your beard look well kempt, all the while complementing your facial structure."

While we are on the subject of hair, nothing says *old man* more than visible nose hair and ear hair. Invest in a good nose and ear hair trimmer, and seek out men-only spas and shops for products and tips on grooming. Men need to pay attention to their eyebrows as well. Just like women, as men get older their hormones change. Whereas women's eyebrows tend to get thinner with age, men's brows may grow thicker and bushier. If your eyebrows are out of control, have your brows professionally trimmed and shaped. There are also special men's eyebrow razors. You can use special scissors to trim long coarse hairs.

Cleaning

As mentioned earlier, if you have not done so recently, it is probably time to clean your closet. That means setting aside time to take everything out—yes everything—as a first step in updating your image. Once you have emptied your closet(s), you need to create and put clothes, shoes, and accessories into five categories:

- Keep
- Keep (alterations needed)

- Sell (eBay or consignment)
- Donate
- Throw away (torn, faded, or too worn)

The best way to determine your categories is to try on each piece and ask yourself the following questions:

- Do I like it?
- Does it fit?
- Is it comfortable?
- Have I worn it within the last three years?
- Will I wear it?
- Do I look good in it?
- Is it in style?
- Do I feel good in it?
- Is it in my color palette?
- Does it reflect my personality?
- Does it reflect my lifestyle?

(Women) When deciding what to do with shoes, consider the following:

- Are they comfortable?
- Are they the right size (width, length)?
- Is the heel height right for me?
- Do they look dated?

Workspace

Maintaining a neat and tidy workspace is important for people, regardless of age. It is even more important for those of us who are older because it communicates a more contemporary image. How you decorate or accessorize your work area will depend on personal preference and workplace *climate*.

In the *old days*, employees were discouraged from making their workspaces look too personal. In fact, some businesses such as banking had specific guidelines for what you could and could not put on your desk or walls. That has all changed because of more people working from home who are used to a personalized work area. Another notable change is shared space and open-space office configurations. In those situations, you are limited in being able to display personal items. Again, observe how younger employees decorate their workspaces. Although your work area should be comfortable and reflect your personality, be careful not to display items that can easily date you such as award plaques or college diplomas, unless they are directly related to your profession.

Take Action!

- Set aside time to clean and organize your clothing closet and drawers.
- Consult a hairstylist about creating a fresh new look.
- Meet with a fashion consultant or personal shopper.
- Make an appointment with a cosmetic dermatologist.

CHAPTER 5

Get Physical

Take care of your body. It's the only place you have to live.
—Jim Rohn, Entrepreneur,
Author, Motivational Speaker

When I started to think about this chapter, two questions came to mind: (1) Where do I start? (2) Where do I stop? The reasons these two questions are so perplexing is because the topic of physical health is complex and overwhelming. There are literally thousands of books, articles, blogs that address health issues as we age. Due to the enormity of the topic, this chapter is meant to serve as a simple reminder of what we can do to slow down the signs of aging by improving and maintaining a healthy lifestyle. The truth is that the healthier we are and continue to be, the more relevant we remain in our fitness and health-conscious society.

Exercise and Physical Activity

A good place to start is with exercise and physical activity. One of the major ways to slow down the aging process is to keep moving. As we age, we tend to slow down and embrace a more sedentary lifestyle. This is a result of bad habits developed over the years and/or health problems that prevent us from remaining physically active. For example, many people over 60 (myself included) suffer from arthritis that takes its toll on joints and prevents or limits us from being as active physically as we have been in the past. We may have difficulty walking or climbing stairs. The cause may be genetics, poor lifestyle, or a combination. Our metabolism starts to decline around age 60. This slowdown is caused by losing muscle and being less active. As a result, the body tends to burn calories at a lower rate. Because your metabolic rate slows, you need fewer calories, yet many of us do not make that adjustment.

If you already engage in physical activity, don't stop just because you have had knee replacements, hip replacements, or ankle and toe fusion. Find what works for you. *Whatever you do, incorporate some type of physical activity into your daily life.* If you don't continue to exercise, your muscles will atrophy. Although sarcopenia, the loss of muscle tissue, is a natural part of aging, we can slow it down. A key point here is that it is never too late to make a lifestyle change. Start by taking a walk around your neighborhood before or after work.

Although the pandemic made it much more difficult to adhere to an exercise program with shuttered gyms and social distancing, there were still ways to get in valuable activity. If you don't have access to exercise equipment such as treadmills or stationary bicycles, in addition to establishing a walking routine, you can buy DVDs or access free YouTube videos and exercise in the comfort and privacy of your home. There are many on the market for folks over 60. If you don't like traditional aerobic exercise, try dancing. Turn on your favorite music and enjoy! If you are traveling by air, take advantage of the waiting time by taking laps around the terminal. Walk around your work site (home or office) while you are on the phone. Unless you really need a handicap spot, park at the farthest spot at the mall or grocery store. The same holds true about taking the stairs if you can rather than the escalator or elevator. Don't forget the benefits of just playing with your dog, children, or grandchildren. The important thing is to MOVE!

As to strength training and multimuscle movement, you can do squats and lunges to work several muscle groups at once. Using inexpensive and very portable equipment such as resistance bands and free weights can work wonders for improving muscle strength and range of motion in addition to speeding up your metabolism, improving your heart rate, and burning calories. Exercise also improves muscle coordination and sharpens your memory. If money is an issue, there are plenty of free resources to help you create your individual exercise program. For example, www.healthline.com presents a suggested weekly exercise plan for older adults complete with video examples of exercises. You can also search YouTube for exercises for older adults. In many cases, motivation is the stumbling block. If so, team up with a friend or family member and hold each other accountable.

Individual or Group

Join the gym or your local YMCA that have exercise programs for active older adults. Group sessions make exercising more fun and interesting. In addition to classes, hire a personal trainer who can tailor an exercise program to your needs and abilities. Your program should consist of a combination of strength training and aerobic exercise. According to Katie Barrett, Director of Fitness at the Union League of Philadelphia, "Classes are great, but you need a personal trainer to tailor a program to your specific goals and physical capabilities. This is particularly important if you have joint issues or have had joint replacements."

"Exercising for Life" (https://aging/exercising-for-life) is a great resource to get you started on an exercise routine. It addresses the benefits of exercise for older adults, what to look for in an exercise routine, and recommended activities for the four aspects of physical health: endurance, balance, strength, and flexibility. As noted in the article, the "American Institute for Cancer Research recommends both physical activity and exercise for a truly healthy lifestyle."

If you are restarting or just beginning your physical fitness program, Katie Barrett acknowledges that "it can be intimidating and overwhelming. The key is to start slowly so you don't get discouraged." She suggests a 30-minute session three or four times a week, alternating between cardio exercise and weight training. She also stresses the importance of making sure to include stretching exercises to improve flexibility as well as exercises to strengthen muscles. One of the biggest mistakes people make with their exercise programs is doing the same routine over and over and not seeing any changes in their weight or body composition. According to Barrett, "Your body gets used to the routine and adapts accordingly so you need to increase weights, volume, and repetitions to get results." This is the reason it is helpful to engage the services of a personal trainer who can guide you along the way.

Mind–Body Connection

Bob Fischer, owner of *i50fit*, located in Southampton, Pennsylvania, is a personal fitness trainer and nutritional counselor, specializing in functional aging and senior fitness. He offers both in-person and virtual, individual and group sessions for people over 50. Following his passion for physical fitness, Bob left his graphic design profession at age 55 to become a personal trainer for active older adults by focusing on functional aging, a combination of the chronological, physiological, mental, and emotional ages. The mission is to help older adults enhance their abilities to function longer in life. Emphasizing the mind–body connection, Bob offers a unique program called "Brains and Balance Past 60." The program is designed to keep active older adults mentally sharp and physically fit by training the brain as we train our skeletal muscles, a topic introduced in Chapter 1, "Stay Sharp." As Bob Fischer puts it, "A stronger body translates to a stronger mind." Studies show exercise and resistance training is the most effective long-term treatment for depression.

This innovative one-hour workshop is divided into four 15-minute segments with alternating balance and brains activities. Balance activities consist of the following:

- Age-appropriate exercises focusing on muscle groups that aid in stability and balance: legs/quads, core/lower abdominals, chest, shoulders, back, hips, and pelvic floor.
- Scenarios that replicate real-life situations: obstacles, uneven surfaces, crowded areas, stairs, sit/stand.
- Modified physical challenges: relay races, kick ball, throwing, hand-eye coordination.

Brain activities involve:

- Memory and cognition challenges: brain teasers, mind benders, puzzles, short-term memory games, math, knowledge, language.
- Small-group problem-solving, card games, concentration exercises, 2D and 3D puzzle building.

Yoga

You may want to incorporate yoga into your exercise regimen. Yoga promotes both physical health as well as mental health, which we will address

in Chapter 6, "Seek Harmony." Here are a few of the physical benefits
of yoga:

- Can lessen lower back pain and headaches
- Can lower blood pressure
- Improves posture and flexibility
- Improves muscle and tone
- Improves blood flow
- Promotes better bone health

Diet and Nutrition

Most of us could do a better job with our eating habits. The importance of following a healthy dietary plan is even more critical as we age.
Again, there are many free resources available online to help you practice
proper nutrition.

Before we address some basics of good nutrition, let us start with
self-awareness and self-assessment as they relate to food. Many of you
might remember the Food Pyramid introduced in 1992 by the U.S.
Department of Agriculture. Its purpose was to help adults understand
what to include in a healthy diet. Since then, the pyramid has undergone
several changes. Most recently, the pyramid concept was replaced in 2011
by MyPlate, a much simpler visual representation. MyPlate is easier to
understand and to follow and is broken down into four unequal sections that represent the different food groups. It also accommodates those
who follow a vegetarian or vegan approach to eating. Visualize your plate
arranged as follows:

- Vegetables—40 percent
- Grains—30 percent
- Protein—20 percent
- Fruits—10 percent
- Dairy—small amounts appearing at the side

This translates into the following quantities based on a 2,000-calorie
daily intake:

Grains	6 ounces
Vegetables	2.5 cups
Fruits	2 cups
Dairy	3 cups
Protein foods	5.5 ounces
Oils	6 teaspoons

Nutrition Checklist

If you want to improve your eating habits and nutrition, start by thinking about your typical weekly food intake and answer *yes* or *no* to the following:

Do you...
- Eat three meals a day?
- Incorporate all USDA MyPlate food groups into your daily diet?
- Follow a plant-based diet?
- Drink at least eight eight-ounce glasses of water a day?
- Stop eating when you are full?
- Eat healthy snacks?
- Avoid eating *on the run*?
- Limit added sugars (less than 10 percent of calories a day)?
- Limit sodium (less than 2,300 milligrams a day)?
- Limit saturated fat (less than 10 percent of calories a day)?

Food Preferences

As we age, our food preferences may not change, but our body's ability to metabolize or react to what we have ingested does change. We may develop food allergies or an intolerance for certain foods or ingredients. For example, when I was younger, I could eat hot chicken wings—the hotter, the better. Those days are long gone! I have come to accept that I cannot eat spicy food that I once craved.

Eating Habits and Weight Management

Habits are hard to break, especially when it comes to eating. We have developed both good and bad eating habits over many years. In many cases, our bad habits have resulted in weight gain and poor nutrition. However, we can break old habits and replace them with new ones. The amount of time depends on the individual and his or her willingness and efforts to change behavior. Here are some tips for improving your eating habits:

- Eat slowly and savor every bite rather than *wolfing it down* to get on to the next thing on your agenda. Take the time to enjoy the eating experience. Use your senses to appreciate the sight, smell, and taste of your meal. Take note of the texture of your food and even the sound when you bite down on your food morsel.
- Practice portion control. The food industry and some restaurants encourage us to eat larger portions so that we perceive we are getting more for our money. Have you noticed how much larger dinner plates are than they were even a few decades ago? If you have any doubt, compare the size of today's dinner plates with those you first bought as an adult. For example, I measured the serving surface diameter of my grandmother's largest dinner plate (6 inches) and compared it to the largest dinner plate serving surface in my dinnerware collection (8 inches). You can certainly pack a lot of food onto those two extra inches!
- Avoid fast-food restaurants and microwavable meals that are high in sodium, even though they may be lower in calories.
- Make good food choices and eat balanced meals by following MyPlate. For a more complete understanding of MyPlate, visit www.ChooseMyPlate.gov and be sure to take the free quiz.
- Ditch the *clean plate club*. Many of us were programmed in our childhood to eat everything on our plates. Instead follow the 80 percent rule. Eat until you are 80 percent full and save the rest for another day.

- Limit your alcohol intake.
- Do not skip meals. Skipping meals throws your body off balance. When you skip a meal, you are more likely to overeat and make poor food choices at your next meal. Make sure you eat three meals a day or several smaller meals throughout the day to keep your body *stoked*.
- Plan your meals. Try to set aside time on Sunday to plan your meals for the week. Ideally, you can both plan the meals and prep them as well. For example, on Sunday, you can cook a chicken to be used in various ways throughout the week, make a pot of soup, or prepare a casserole, all of which require you to heat and serve.

Water

The importance of drinking water at any age cannot be overstated. However, it's even more critical for older adults. According to research published in the *Journal of Gerontology Nursing*, between 20 and 30 percent of older adults are chronically dehydrated. Like other changes as our bodies age, our sense of thirst decreases as does the amount of water we have stored in our bodies, but our need for water does not. It is commonly recommended that people drink eight eight-ounce glasses of water per day in addition to eating foods that provide additional fluid intake. Staying hydrated is important for several reasons. Our body needs water to help regulate body temperature, lubricate joints, excrete waste, prevent constipation, aid digestion, maintain muscle strength, and boost metabolism, among many other functions.

Water can also help weight management. Often when we feel hungry, what the body really needs is water. So, before you grab that mid-afternoon snack, pour a glass of water instead. Your feeling of hunger will most likely go away. Also, if you experience symptoms of mild dehydration (headache, fatigue, and difficulty concentrating) between meals, drink some water and notice how quickly you perk up.

Tips for Staying Hydrated

- Keep a reusable bottle of water with you and drink throughout the day.
- Add a slice of cucumber, lemon, or other fruit to your water to make it more interesting and satisfying.
- Set a timer on your phone to remind you to drink water.
- Eat foods high in water content such as fruits, vegetables, and soups.
- Drink water with every meal.
- Drink water before and after exercise.
- Reduce alcohol intake.
- Monitor the color of your urine. Dark or colored urine indicates dehydration.

Posture

There is a good reason your mother told you to *stand up straight* and *don't slouch*. Years of bad posture may have created rounded shoulders, that is, when shoulders are out of proper alignment with the spine, now compounded by the number of hours we spend using the computer, driving a car, sitting for long periods, or bending over repeatedly. Not only do we experience pain, but we also look old and hunched over. If you fall into this category, see a physician, chiropractor, or physical therapist.

Women, in particular, exhibit signs of poor body alignment caused by years of wearing high heels. I remember a manager I had when I was in my 30s saying to a colleague and me, "You, girls, one of these days you're going to regret wearing those high heels." Behind her back, we rolled our eyes, dismissed her warning, and vowed to never give up our heels. The day of reckoning has arrived! This was good advice then, and it is good advice now.

When you see someone with rounded shoulders and bent over, subconsciously, you conclude that this person is old. Although it is true, that both men and women lose height as they age (starting at around age 30), loss of height becomes more pronounced after age 70. The wear and tear on the musculoskeletal system (bones, muscles, and joints) over the years can have a profound effect on our posture. Loss of bone density results in osteoporosis. In addition to loss of calcium to the bones, intervertebral discs lose their flexibility, and these changes that are all a normal part of aging cause a formal tilt called kyphosis. Kyphosis is a spinal disorder in which an excessive outward curve of the spine creates an abnormal rounding of the upper back. This condition is most common in older women and is often related to osteoporosis.

Muscle mass also changes with age and can contribute to curvature of the spine. Another factor that influences stature is the change from a lean body to one with more fat, especially around the waist. This change in weight also contributes to changes in the spine.

We cannot prevent these changes, but we can slow them down or minimize them. The most important strategy is exercise because it improves bone and muscle toning. The more you exercise, the more your posture will improve. A proper and balanced diet can also improve your overall health. It is also important to supplement a healthy diet with calcium and vitamin D found in dairy products, fatty fish, and some cereals.

While age-related changes certainly contribute to posture problems, many back problems are a result of bad habits we have developed over the years. According to Dr. David Binder of the Orthopedic Spine Center at Harvard-affiliated Massachusetts General Hospital, "Healthy posture depends on the right movements and alignments of your hips, spine, neck, and jaw, as well as surrounding muscles that offer support."

Poor posture can also contribute to falls and poor balance. It affects how well your heart can pump blood and how well you breathe. If you have any doubts, conduct your own experiment. Sit in a chair and slump forward. Now take a breath and note how deeply you can breathe. Then sit up and back in the chair with your head up and shoulders down. In your sitting tall position, take a deep breath and notice the difference. Recent studies find that people with better posture are healthier and live longer.

The following tips and techniques can help you improve and maintain your posture:

- *See a physical therapist.* Because everyone is different, it's a good idea to get a referral to see a physical therapist who can determine the best posture for you.
- *Get up and move.* If you have a job that requires you to sit or stand for long periods, it is critical that you move around at least every 20 minutes. According to Dr. David Binder, "This helps to reduce muscle fatigue and muscle strain that leads to slouching."
- *Get your vision checked.* Going for an eye exam once a year is just one of the many body maintenance appointments you must do. In addition to making sure you can see and getting fitted for the proper glasses or contact lenses to improve your vision, you will be helping your posture as well. Poor eyesight can cause you to push your head forward to read or to see the television or computer screen.
- *Practice yoga or tai chi.* Exercises such as yoga or tai chi involve movements and positions that improve posture. These exercises have many other benefits as well.

Dr. Steven Weiniger, a posture expert and author of *Stand Taller— Live Longer: An Anti-Aging Strategy,* suggests the one-leg balance exercise three times a day to help improve your balance.

- Stand up, tall and straight.
- Lift your left leg so your thigh is level with the ground.
- Count to 20.
- Repeat on the other side.

Sleep

Another change as we age is our sleep patterns such as comfortable temperature, body position, and amount of sleep. Studies have shown that getting enough sleep prevents illness such as high blood pressure and stroke. Furthermore, lack of sleep has been linked to obesity, heart disease, Type 2 diabetes, and depression, among others.

To get a picture of your sleep habits, respond to the following:

Sleep Habits Assessment

In the past month, have you experienced...?
- Difficulty going to sleep?
- Waking up in the middle of the night?
- Getting fewer than six hours of sleep a night?
- Bad dreams?
- Pain?
- Snoring?
- Getting up in the middle of the night to go to the bathroom?
- Feeling tired the next day?
- Difficulty breathing?
- Taking medications to help you sleep?
- Difficulty staying awake during the day?

If you answered *yes* to even a few of these questions, you need to see your health care professional. In the meantime, here are some tips from professionals to help improve your sleep habits:

- Avoid cigarettes.
- Drink alcohol in moderation.
- Eat dinner at the same time every evening.
- Go to bed and get up at the same time every day, even on weekends.
- Do not exercise too close to bedtime.
- Turn off the lights and sleep in a darkened bedroom.
- Do not use electronic devices while you are in bed.
- Use a cooling blanket or weighted blanket depending on your preference.
- Use white noise, a sound machine, relaxing music to block out extraneous noise and help you fall asleep.

- Drink soothing tea before going to bed.
- Replace your mattress after 10 years and your pillow every 1–2 years.

Skin

So many people in the over-60 category have done major damage to their skin over the years beginning in their teens by dousing their bodies with baby oil and lying in the scorching sun to get that perfect tan. Sunscreen was unheard of until the late 1980s and early 1990s. By that time, the damage was done; however, experts tell us that there are some steps you can take to mitigate the impact of those UV (ultraviolet) rays.

Sun Exposure

You can still enjoy outdoor activities in the sun, even on the beach, by taking preventive measures. Start by wearing broad spectrum sunscreen (SPF 30 or more), and reapply at least every 80 minutes and wear a hat. Better yet, sit in the shade. In general, limit your time in the sun to early morning (before 10:00) or late afternoon (after 2:00) when the sun is less intense. This, of course, depends on the time of year and your location. If you live in or travel to a warm climate, you need to take extra precautions to guard against sun exposure and damage all year round. Also, be sure to wear sunglasses that protect your eyes. More about that later in this chapter.

Skin Care

As we age, our skin becomes drier, rougher, less firm, and loses elasticity. As discussed in Chapter 4, "Update Your Image," your skin appearance is an important factor in maintaining a youthful appearance. Dry, itchy skin, wrinkles, age spots, and skintags are associated with aging. As noted in Chapter 4, dermatologists can help with cosmetic treatments such as chemical peels, microdermabrasion, laser therapy, beta-carotene, or retinoids. From a physiological perspective, here are some skin care guidelines to help you look and feel your best:

- *Hydrate.* As noted in the section on "Water," staying hydrated by drinking plenty of fluids daily can help promote healthy skin and replenish moisture due to aging.
- *Cleanse.* When bathing, use warm, not hot, water. Hot water strips skin of moisture. Also, use a soft washcloth instead of a loofah or buff puff that can irritate your skin.
- *Moisturize.* Immediately following your shower or bath, apply moisturizer especially for dry skin and exposed areas through-out the day.
- *Exfoliate.* Exfoliate to remove dry skin cells that make your skin look old. Use a buffered glycolic acid-containing cream that gently exfoliates as well as hydrates. Do some research to find the right product for you or ask your dermatologist for a recommendation.
- *Monitor.* Visit your dermatologist annually for a full body skin exam. In between visits, keep a watchful eye for any changes in moles, birthmarks, or other unusual growths such as actinic keratosis. These scaly, crusty patches are a result of sun damage, and without treatment, they may turn into skin cancer. Skin cancer can be cured if caught early.

Mouth and Teeth

Like the other parts of your body, the oral cavity is amazing. Yet the years of grinding, chomping, gnawing, eating acidic foods, and skipping annual dental checkups may have taken their toll. Studies show that people over 65 are more likely to have gum disease, cavities, mouth infections, oral cancer, and tooth loss. You may not be able to reverse the damage that is already done, but you can take steps to keep your mouth looking and feeling younger.

- Practice basic oral hygiene by brushing your teeth and flossing at least twice a day.
- Get regular cleanings and checkups as recommended by your dentist.
- Ask your dentist about using whitening products to remove stains and discoloration.

- Use mouthwash daily.
- Drink water, chew sugarless gum, or suck on sugarless candy to moisten a dry mouth.
- Eat healthy foods and limit sugar intake.
- If you smoke, stop!

Eyes

Have you noticed that the print on labels, prescription bottles, menus, and even the newspaper seem to have gotten smaller? While that may be true in some cases, it's quite likely your eyesight is not as good as it used to be. Like it or not, changes in vision are part of the aging process.

Common Changes

Presbyopia is characterized by difficulty focusing on objects close up such as trouble reading small print. This is normally corrected with eyeglasses or contact lenses.

Floaters appear as spots or threads that drift around in your eye. They are annoying but basically harmless. If, however, you notice many floaters all at once, it could be an indicator of something more serious such as a detached retina. If this happens, seek medical attention immediately.

Dry eyes can be caused by allergies, medications, contact lenses, or Lasik eye surgery resulting in burning, scratchy, watery eyes, and blurred vision. Eye drops such as Refresh, Vision Tears, Blink, or Systane can help.

In addition to these common changes, eyes are often prone to age-related diseases. If left untreated, you could lose your vision entirely.

Critical Eye Diseases

Cataracts

Cataracts develop slowly over time and are characterized by visible cloudiness and blurred vision. Night-time driving may become particularly troublesome due to light sensitivity, double vision, or seeing halos.

Macular Degeneration

Macular degeneration is a thinning of the *macula*, which is part of the retina that makes vision clear and details. Although it is incurable, there are varying degrees of severity, but all involve some degree of vision loss.

Glaucoma

Glaucoma is a condition when the optic nerve becomes damaged and can lead to sudden and complete loss of vision. The damage is irreversible.

Diabetic Eye Disease

Diabetic eye disease, also called diabetic retinopathy, occurs when the blood vessels of the retina are damaged. People with diabetes need to monitor their blood pressure and blood sugar carefully. Left untreated, it could result in blindness.

Eye Care

Not surprising, the guidelines for taking care of your eyes are much the same as those for our general health such as exercise, good nutrition (especially foods rich in vitamin C and antioxidants), adequate sleep, smoking cessation, and annual checkups with your health care professional. In addition, make sure you have good indoor lighting and reduce eye strain from working on your computer or watching television by taking a 20–30-second break every 20 minutes.

Not only are eyes "the window to the soul," they are also the window to our world, and they need to be protected. According to the American Academy of Ophthalmology, "Excess sun exposure can put you at risk for eye cancer, sunburned eyes, cataracts, and growths on or near the eye." It can also worsen macular degeneration. One way to protect your eyes is by wearing proper sunglasses when outdoors, sun or clouds, all year round. In addition to being functional, sunglasses are an important accessory for the fashion-conscious, and for that reason, many of us gravitate to the designer brands and/or the inexpensive drugstore versions. Most of these are not going to protect your eyes. Rest assured that you can still look *in* and fashionable without leaving your eyes vulnerable to those damaging UV rays. When choosing sunglasses, consider the following guidelines:

- Lenses that block 99 to 100 percent of both UVA and UVB rays or are labeled UV400
- Oversized lenses and wrap around styles that will protect more area
- Polarized lenses to reduce glare from water, snow, pavement
- Wider temples that block even more UV light
- Personal preference as to color and darkness of lenses

Potential Warning Signs

Please make an appointment with your eye care professional if you experience any of the following:

- Double vision
- Light sensitivity
- Seeing halos
- Blurred vision
- Difficulty seeing at a distance
- Difficulty reading
- Loss of peripheral vision
- Eye pain
- Flashing lights in your vision
- Excessive floaters
- Poor or diminished perception of color

Ears

Our ears are an integral part of our physical, emotional, and psychological well-being. They help us relate to the world around us. Our ears enable us to hear, and hearing connects us to information and to people. This ability to be engaged helps us remain relevant, so it is incumbent on us to take good care of the vehicle we have been given to connect with people and our surroundings.

Hearing Loss

Hearing loss can happen at any age and for a variety of reasons. It is, however, associated with the aging process. Age-related hearing loss may come on gradually and, therefore, be ignored until it becomes an issue impacting your quality of life. To many, there is a stigma attached to hearing loss. They associate it with being old. These same people may have no problem getting fitted for contact lenses or glasses to correct their failing eyesight, but they become resistant to getting a hearing aid. Ignoring your hearing loss can negatively impact your social, emotional, and psychological well-being. It can also adversely affect your job and interactions with others, giving credence to the perception that you are old and not relevant. It is time to seek the professional help of a hearing specialist when you experience these warning signs:

- Difficulty hearing conversations
- Inability to block out background noise
- Needing the volume on the television or radio to be louder
- Difficulty hearing some environmental sounds
- Asking people to repeat what they have said
- Answer inappropriately because you misunderstood what the person said
- Difficulty hearing on the telephone
- Think other people are mumbling
- Withdrawing from conversations
- People telling you to get your hearing tested

If you need a hearing aid, swallow your pride, research options, choose the right product and provider, then just do it! You will be glad you did and wonder why you waited so long. If you have a complete hearing loss, you have many options available to help you continue to be productive and relevant.

Wax Buildup

Earwax is a substance called cerumen that binds dirt, debris, dust, and tiny hairs, produced by the body, to cleanse, lubricate, and protect our ears. Although earwax buildup can occur at any stage of life, it tends to increase with age. Like many other parts of our body, this natural lubricant becomes drier. As a result, it becomes harder and moves more slowly out of the canal causing a buildup over time. This accumulation of earwax creates a blockage and may cause hearing loss, ringing, or a feeling of fullness in the ear. People who wear hearing aids are more prone to earwax blockage.

To keep earwax under control, gently clean your ears each day by wiping around your ear with a damp washcloth on your finger. Do not insert Q-tips or any other objects in your ears! To remove earwax yourself, you can use a softening agent, baby oil or mineral oil, or an over-the-counter product such as Debrox Earwax Removal Kit.

If these methods don't work, it's time to seek medical help starting with your primary care physician. He or she will use one of two methods: (1) scooping it out with a special instrument or (2) sending a force of water via an irrigation device. If the ear is really impacted, you will need to see an otolaryngologist who will use specialty tools to dislodge the wax.

Hands and Feet

Over the years, our appendages have taken a beating, especially our feet. Although some hand and foot problems are out of our control such as arthritis, there are also some actions we can take to correct some of the damage already done.

Foot Care

When your feet hurt, you hurt all over. Be kind to your feet, and they will be kind to you. Over time, the fatty padding in our feet wears down, leaving them more vulnerable to bone and joint wear and tear. Your feet become more sensitive to external stimuli such as heat, cold, and objects that may cause pain. If you have any doubt, observe younger folks walking barefoot on hot pavement in the middle of a hot summer day.

Neglecting your feet may lead to serious problems that not only cause pain but also impact your quality of life. If you have trouble walking because of foot problems, you will be limited in your ability to participate in social activities or physical activities such as walking and exercising. This becomes a downward spiral that can affect your entire well-being. Here are some tips to help you maintain healthy and happy feet:

- *Clean.* Just as you do with the rest of your body, keep your feet clean to prevent infections. This includes making sure you dry your feet thoroughly after washing them.
- *Moisturize.* As noted earlier, skin becomes drier with age. After washing and drying your feet, lock in that moisture with a good foot lotion.
- *Trim.* Keep your nails trimmed to prevent foot-related problems. If you can't or don't want to deal with this yourself, make appointments for monthly pedicures or seek the services of a podiatrist.
- *Massage.* A foot massage can work wonders for both body and spirit. In addition to just feeling good, massaging your feet aids circulation, stimulates muscles, reduces tension, and sometimes relieves pain. A foot massage is generally included in a spa treatment or pedicure. If you prefer the do-it-yourself route that you can do routinely, there are many electric foot massagers on the market.
- *Monitor.* Keep a careful watch on your feet for signs of bunions, hammer toes, corns, calluses, discolored toenails, ingrown toenails, or blisters. Other more serious conditions such as diabetic neuropathy (nerve damage) or plantar fasciitis (an inflammation) *cry out* for treatment. If so, you need to make an appointment with a health care professional. In some cases, you may be able to deal with these conditions on your own but most likely home treatments will be in conjunction with a doctor's recommendations.
- *Cool.* After torturing your feet by taking a long walk or stand-ing all day, it just feels good to cool your feet. Try ice pack slippers. These are great even if you just want to cool your feet on a hot day. More importantly, the handy, inexpensive

gel-filled slippers mold to the bottom of your feet and help reduce inflammation and swelling from plantar fasciitis and spurs or ease arthritis toe pain.

These foot care tips apply to both men and women. If you do not address foot issues, they will only get worse. I discovered that the hard way. I was in a great deal of pain in my right foot and had difficulty walking no matter what shoe I was wearing. After seeing an orthopedic surgeon, I was told that because of arthritis, I had no cartilage in my right big toe and needed a *big toe* fusion along with the removal of a bone spur associated with it. I delayed having the surgery because the surgeon told me that I would not be able to wear heels again. Talk about vanity and stupidity! I was not a candidate for a less-invasive procedure because I waited too long.

Footwear

In addition to the damage high heels cause with body alignment mentioned earlier, they wreak havoc on our feet. As my orthopedic surgeon, Dr. Kathryn O'Connor, a specialist in foot and ankle problems, said when I showed up for an appointment wearing cute ballet flats, "If it's really cute, it's probably not good for your feet." You don't have to sacrifice fashion for comfort and good foot care. You may have to do some research, but there are a lot of shoes on the market that meet the following criteria for *sensible* (orthopedic specialist and podiatrist-approved), yet fashionable, shoes:

- Good arch support. That eliminates ballet flats and many sandals, especially flip flops.
- Proper length and width. Our feet lengthen and flatten with age, especially with pregnancy and weight gain. You may need a half size larger or a wider shoe. Don't try to squeeze your foot into a shoe that is too small.
- Plenty of room for your toes. That eliminates pointed toes.
- Reasonable heel height—no higher than 2 inches.

Although much of what I just presented is targeted to women, some men fall into the same trap of wearing shoes that are too short or too narrow and the wrong shape. Have your feet measured by a sales professional at a quality shoe specialty store.

Hand Care

Although the basics of hand care are much the same as those for foot care and skin care, there are some distinct differences. Just like your feet, hands lose fat. They also lose elasticity, and your skin loses volume. This results in noticeable veins, wrinkly skin, age spots, and thin, bony hands. To regain some of that lost youthful fullness, consult a dermatologist. Many treatments such as fillers, your own fat, laser therapy, chemical peeling, cryotherapy (freezing), microdermabrasion, creams, and lotions can help rejuvenate your hands. At the very least, you need to do the following:

- *Moisturize.* Use hand lotion throughout the day and especially after you wash your hands. Be sure to rub the lotion into your fingernails and cuticles, too.
- *Protect.* In addition to using sunscreen to protect your hands from the sun, you need to wear gloves to protect them when you are cleaning or doing yard work.
- *Exfoliate.* Just as the rest of your body needs exfoliating, so do your hands to remove dead skin and dead skin cells.
- *Monitor.* Keep a close eye out for any changes in your hands and nails. These includes changes in color, texture, shape, and general appearance. Be on the lookout for changes to the shape of your fingers. Hard bony lumps in the joints of your fingers may be a symptom of osteoarthritis and should prompt you to make an appointment with your primary care physician who may refer you to a rheumatologist.

Chronological Versus Biological Age

People have two ages: biological and chronological. Chronological age refers to the actual number of years you have been alive. Unfortunately, this is what most people focus on. On the other hand, our biological age is based on a combination of environmental/lifestyle factors such as diet, exercise, sleeping habits, stress, alcohol consumption, and smoking. Your biological age is how well or how poorly your body is functioning relative to your chronological age. For a reflection of how well your body is aging, access an online biological age calculator (www.biological-age.com) or (www.easycalculation.com/health/biological-age.php).

When people *seem* younger than their chronological age, it is because they maintain a healthy lifestyle and eliminate metabolic imbalances (toxins and allergens) in their bodies. This anti-aging approach is practiced by Dr. Robert Brookman, a leading national expert in anti-aging, regenerative, and functional medicine. Based in Philadelphia, Pennsylvania, Dr. Brookman emphasizes the importance of looking at a multitude of "inter-related physiological processes and pathologies that must be considered in order to promote a total well-being."

Personal Health Maintenance

If you have (or had) a car, you probably take it to a garage or repair shop for routine maintenance to ensure it remains in good running condition. Often, you are prompted by warning lights, sounds, or electronic dashboard messages. If you decide to ignore those alerts, the vehicle you rely on to transport you to work, help you run errands, and shuttle you to social events may break down, resulting in costly repairs. The same holds true for our body that sends out signals when it needs attention or is in distress. Shouldn't we maintain our bodies even more than we maintain our cars? Failure to act can lead to a variety of illnesses and diseases that perhaps could have been prevented. Think about this: when your car wears out, you can get another one; when your body wears out, it can be the end of the road.

Personal Health Maintenance Checklist

To help get a clearer picture of your personal health maintenance, refer to your calendar and/or medical records and answer the following:

When was the last time you had a(an)…?

- Complete physical exam?
- Dental checkup and cleaning?
- Eye exam?
- Hearing test?
- Full body skin exam?
- Colon cancer screening?
- (Women) Mammogram?

If you cannot remember or if it has been well over a year, you probably need to make appointments with your health care professionals starting with your primary care physician. Keep in mind that the first available appointments may be months away.

Making the Case for a Healthy Lifestyle

One of the major benefits I have received from writing this book is what I have learned from the people I interviewed. During our interview and our discussion of health and aging, Dr. Gary Dorshimer talked about the regions in the world where people live the longest and what the inhabitants do that contribute to their longevity as well as the mental and physical benefits to themselves and their societies. The five regions are addressed in the book *The Blue Zones: Lessons for Living Longer from the People Who've Lived the Longest* and include Sardinia, Italy; Okinawa, Japan; Nicoya Peninsula, Costa Rica; Icaria, Greece, and a community of Seventh-day Adventists in Loma Linda, California. Interestingly and unknowingly, I addressed their lifestyle practices in three of this book's chapters:

Get physical	Moderate, regular physical activity; moderate caloric intake; plant-based diet; moderate alcohol intake
Seek harmony	Life purpose; stress reduction; engagement in spirituality or religion
Stay connected	Engagement in family life; engagement in social life

Think about it. By practicing a healthy lifestyle, you can live a long life well past the traditional retirement age. That means another 30 plus years to remain relevant and continue to be a contributing member of society.

Take Action!

- Start or upgrade your exercise/physical fitness program.
- Make appointments with your health care professionals for appropriate checkups/evaluations.
- Calculate your biological age and compare it to your chronological age. Identify areas where you want/need to improve.

CHAPTER 6

Seek Harmony

You cannot always control what goes on outside. But you can always control what goes on inside.

—Dr. Wayne Dyer, American
Self-Help Author and Motivational Speaker

In addition to our physical being, mind and spirit play a significant role in helping us remain relevant. The spiritual, psychological, and emotional aspects of our lives contribute to a mindset—positive or negative—that impacts behavior. In this chapter, we will focus on ways to relieve stress, maintain a positive self-image, and overcome internal obstacles that undermine our efforts to remain relevant.

It may seem strange to begin a chapter that advocates seeking harmony with a discussion about stress, but the more we can understand stress, the better we will be at mobilizing all our resources to minimize stress and experience the harmony we seek. Notice I said minimize, not eliminate. Stress is unavoidable; it is a part of life. In fact, we need a certain degree of stress in our daily lives. Too much stress causes frustration; too little stress results in boredom. In and of itself, stress is neither good nor bad. Our own personal reaction to stress creates either positive or negative results.

Although stress is often exacerbated by major and sometimes catastrophic events, whether they be personal (death of a family member, loss of income, personal health issues, work-related pressures) or more global (pandemic, war, natural disasters), it is how we respond to those events that determines strength of character. When I was growing up and *bad things* happened to me (getting a bad grade, being dumped by my boyfriend, or having *zits* on my face), my mother would always say, "It builds character." As I got older and the *bad things* were more serious, my retort to her was, "I have had enough character building." Of course, the reality is that life is a continuous character-building process.

Understanding Stress

Every day we deal with stressors in our personal and professional lives. Everyday demands and pressures—too much to do and too little time—can take their toll. Stressors are those external events that can cause physical and psychological reaction. These stressors trigger a real or perceived threat. Different people react differently to stressful situations. Perception is the determining factor in the extent to which any one stressor affects a particular individual. The problem with stress is that it is cumulative.

The sources of stress change over our lifetime (balancing family, career, and sometimes school). If you have children, most likely they are now grown and have families of their own. That creates a whole separate set of stressors.

Before we get into examining stress in more detail, take a moment to assess your own stress level by responding to the following self-assessment:

Stress Self-Assessment

Instructions: Using the following key, indicate how often during the past six months you have experienced the following:

KEY: 5—Frequently (90%); 4—Often (70%); 3—Sometimes (50%); 2—Seldom (30%); 1—Never (0%)

1. Changes in sleep patterns, that is, sleeping more or less.
2. Increased use of alcohol, prescription drugs, cigarettes, or caffeine.
3. Physical pains such as headaches, muscle aches, and backaches.
4. Difficulty concentrating or focusing on tasks; forgetfulness.
5. Decreased productivity and quality of work.
6. Lack of interest in job or activities you once enjoyed.
7. Problems expressing your feelings or thoughts to family members, friends, or colleagues.
8. More frequent colds or allergy *flare ups.*

9. Emotional outbursts; increased irritability and argumentative behavior.

10. Feelings of hopelessness and despair.

11. Difficulty making decisions.

12. Tendency to spend more time alone or engage in escapist activities such as watching television.

13. Feeling alone and isolated, even when you are with other people.

14. Change in eating behaviors, that is, eating more or less.

15. Digestive problems such as diarrhea, constipation, nausea, heartburn.

16. Lack of energy; tiredness, fatigue.

17. Feeling overwhelmed and immobilized.

18. More critical, less tolerant of other people.

19. Lack of physical and/or emotional intimacy.

20. Engaging in habits such as foot tapping, nail biting, finger drumming, or teeth grinding.

Total:

Interpretation:

20–28   Your life is stress-free! Congratulations!

29–45   Your stress level is fairly normal, especially given these trying times.

46–74   Your stress level is higher than normal. You need to begin practicing stress reduction techniques.

75–91   Your stress level is cause for concern. Make stress management a priority.

92–100 Your stress level could lead to serious medical problems. Seek professional help.

Increasing Self-Awareness

The purpose of a self-assessment is to increase your awareness and understanding of the behaviors that may be keeping you from being as effective as you would like to be. Review your overall self-assessment total as well as specific items that caught your attention. Then answer the following questions:

- What is your reaction to your self-assessment? How did you feel about completing it?
- What did you learn about yourself? What insights did you gain?
- How can these insights be helpful to you, both professionally and personally?

Self-Assessment: What Do I Value?

As part of the increasing self-awareness process, it is also helpful to look at your values.

Instructions: Please rank the following values in order of their importance to you, with 1 being the most important value and 14 the least important value.

_____ **Knowledge and Wisdom**
To learn new things and ideas; personal growth through experience.

_____ **Morality and Ethics**
To maintain a sense of right and wrong and personal integrity; to adhere to commonly accepted standards or code of conduct.

_____ **Freedom and Independence**
To be able to make own decisions and use own judgment; sense of personal empowerment.

_____ **Love and Affection**
To experience a sense of caring for and from other people.

_____ **Money and Security**
To have enough income and resources to provide for wants and needs; to feel safe in your environment.

_____ **Mental and Physical Health**
To be free of stress, anxiety, and physical illness; to be fit and energetic.

_____ **Religious Beliefs and Spirituality**
To believe in a supreme being or spiritual force.

_____ **Friendship and Relationships**
To have a sense of belonging to a person or group; companionship.

_____ **Pleasure and Enjoyment**
To participate in things you like to do; to have fun and enjoy life; to actively pursue balance and variety in your life.

_____ **Achievement and Accomplishment**
To have a feeling of self-satisfaction as a result of completing a task, overcoming an obstacle, or meeting a challenge; accomplishing goals.

_____ **Loyalty and Trust**
To experience a feeling of dedication and commitment to friends, family, country, organization, and so forth; to have confidence in the integrity and honesty of others.

_____ **Power and Influence**
To have a sense of control and influence over yourself and others.

_____ **Justice and Equity**
To believe in a system that rewards positive behavior and punishes negative behavior; sense of fairness.

_____ **Respect and Civility**
To value and appreciate others; to be considerate and courteous.

Living Your Values

After completing your values self-assessment, review your top six, and then ask yourself the following questions:

- What is my behavior that supports that value?
- What is my behavior that contradicts that value?
- What is the personal impact when my behavior is not congruent with my values?
- What changes do I need to make in my behavior so that I am congruent with my values?

Life Wheel

Another useful tool and exercise for assessing how balanced your life currently is and providing the harmony you seek is the Life Wheel originally developed by Paul J. Meyer, founder of the Success Motivation Institute in 1960. Although there are many versions and adaptations, the basic theory behind the Life Wheel is that our lives consist of certain categories. The number of categories range from six to 10 depending on the author. For our purposes, I have created a Life Wheel with eight categories:

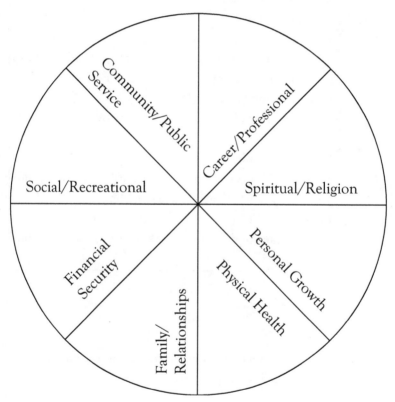

Figure 6.1 Life wheel

To gain a better understanding of what you should include in each of the life wheel categories, consider the following descriptions:

Table 6.1 Life wheel descriptions

Category	Explanation	Examples
Career/Professional	Refers to not only your current job but what you want to do professionally in the long term	Work environment Work hours Meaning/purpose
Spiritual/Religion	Refers to formal religious activities or to anything of a spiritual nature	Meditation Religious attendance
Personal Growth	Refers to activities that engage your mind, such as nonrecreational reading or specific, intellectually stimulating endeavors	Learning Education Reading
Physical Health	Refers to all aspects of your physical being	Exercise Sleep Nutrition Relaxation
Family/Relationships	Refers to the amount of time and attention you devote to those closest to you	Closeness Intimacy Spouse/partner Children Parents/siblings Other relatives
Financial Security	Refers to your current financial requirements and behaviors as well as your future financial needs and concerns	Savings Financial planning Investing Budgeting Housing
Social/Recreational	Refers to activities you might engage in with others or just spending time by yourself	Hobbies Friends Group get-togethers Vacation
Community/Public Service	Refers to activities directed at improving your community and the world around you	Volunteering Charities

Activity: Create Your Life Wheel

1. Start by looking at the preceding *balanced* wheel. Although each of the sections is the same size, the reality is that each person's wheel will be different depending on his or her situation.
2. Next, draw your wheel as it is today, keeping in mind all eight sections. Think about how much time, energy, and effort you devote to

each life category and then draw the appropriate-size wedge. Your estimate is purely subjective. Some categories may not even appear on your *real* wheel, and some may be depicted as mere slivers.

3. Now draw your *ideal* wheel, that is, draw your life wheel as you would like it to be.

Are your *real* wheel and *ideal* wheel in sync or closely matched? If they are, that's great! What if they are not similar? If they are particularly far apart, the result is stress. So, what can you do about it? Carefully examine your life wheel sections and determine which ones you want to bring closer to your ideal state. Then, set specific goals and action plans to bring them into balance and reduce your stress. We will address goal setting and action plans in Chapter 8, "Reinvent Yourself."

I was conducting a seminar on "Managing Priorities and Stress" for an investment firm on Wall Street. One of the participants, John, looked and acted very stressed. After completing his Life Wheel, it became clear to him why he was so stressed. He was in his late 20s, married with two young children. He made a lot of money, lived in a big house on Long Island, and drove an expensive SUV. He seemed to have it all, but he was miserable! His job required him to work long hours, and his commute between Long Island and Lower Manhattan was taking its toll on him personally and professionally.

He left the house early in the morning before the children got up and arrived home after they were in bed. He spent little time with the family even on weekends. His marriage was suffering, and that impacted his job performance. He knew he needed to do something and hoped that the seminar would help him, and it did. He set some specific goals and took action to bring his Real Life Wheel and his Ideal Life Wheel more in sync.

He set a goal to increase the amount and quality of time he spent with his family. One of the action items was to have a date night with his wife once a month. He would make all the arrangements (babysitter, dinner reservations, tickets, and so forth).

I saw John three months later in a follow-up session. He was a changed man. By that time, he and his wife had had three date nights, and she was happy not only because of the outings but also because he took responsibility for making them happen. The improvement in his personal life transferred to his professional life as well. He was happier and more productive at work.

Keep in mind that a balanced wheel is different for each person and will change over your lifetime. Your wheels are going to look different based on where you are on your life's journey. Depending on your circumstances, you may be able to accept the out-of-balance wheel because you know it is not going to last forever. For example, when I was working on my doctorate, running a business, donating a lot of time and effort to professional organizations, my wheel was way out of balance, and I was very stressed. However, I was willing to accept it because I knew the amount of time and effort I was devoting to the *personal growth* category would soon change once I finished my degree.

Symptoms of Stress

First, how do you recognize stress? What are the symptoms? The most common physical symptoms can include digestive problems, muscle aches, fatigue, colds, headaches, and pounding heart.

Behavior changes such as the increased use of drugs, alcohol, or cigarettes are also warning signs. Emotional outbursts, mood swings, irritability, depression, anxiety, frustration, lethargy, and expressions of inadequacy and low self-esteem are all symptoms of stress exhaustion. A change in eating habits resulting in weight gain or loss can also be a symptom. A person on the verge of stress exhaustion will experience reduced clarity of judgment, forgetfulness, poor concentration, confusion, dull senses, and low productivity.

Relationships with others will be affected. If you notice yourself becoming less tolerant of others' behaviors and wonder why, the answer could be stress. Those who are normally outgoing may become withdrawn and clam up. Sometimes an otherwise mild-mannered person might lash out for no apparent reason. The point is that any marked behavior change should be suspect. Untreated, stress will lead to hypertension, heart attacks, severe ulcers, and even death.

Causes of Stress

Before you can begin to deal with stress, it's important to have a clear understanding of the underlying causes. One of the biggest contributors to stress and subsequent burnout is the perception of lack of personal control. Employees in demoralizing work situations will experience increased stress symptoms. In today's demanding environment, the most obvious cause is work overload. However, there are other factors that contribute to stress as well.

- Jobs that have high demand, low control, and allow little latitude for decision making appear to be more stress producing.
- An overly critical boss can create stress.
- Lack of information and communication can also lead to stress.
- People who do not understand their specific job responsibilities, have no sense of direction, or receive little or no recognition will be stressed.
- A lack of clarity regarding policies and procedures or organizational philosophy and mission is stressful for employees.
- Change is a source of great stress. That is why, stress levels increase during mergers and reorganizations.
- Ambiguity coupled with lack of control often results in negative behaviors.

Associated Conditions

Many people often confuse stress, anxiety, and worry. Although they are related, they are not the same, and it is important to know the difference.

Worry

Worry is something that happens in the mind and is future oriented. People who worry have repetitive, obsessive, negative thoughts that focus on uncertain outcomes and things that could go wrong. Worry can be positive when it prompts us to problem-solve or to take action. One effective way to deal with worries is to write them down. Studies have shown that writing them down can help calm obsessive thoughts. You may even want to formalize the process by creating a worry box or engaging the services of a Worry Eater. Worry Eaters are soft plush toys that come in different shapes and sizes. They were created to help children cope with their worries, fears, and troubles. Each Worry Eater has a zippered mouth. The child writes down (or draws) his or her trouble on a piece of paper, puts it in the toy's mouth, zips it shut, and now the Worry Eater takes care of it. The message that comes with the toy states, "I'm (toy's name), and I take care of your worries so you don't have to." It may seem like a silly thing for an adult to do, but an adult participant in one of my stress management sessions admitted that she uses it and suggested it for her worried colleagues.

Another effective way to manage worry is to schedule worry time. Set aside 15 to 30 minutes a day at the same time each day to cope with your worries. During this period, you will focus on problem-solving and developing an action plan to address your worries.

Anxiety

Anxiety is the culmination of stress and worry. As already discussed, worry is cognitive, and stress is a physiological response to a real threat. Anxiety is both a cognitive and a physiological response to a perceived threat. Talking or thinking about your anxiety will not help. The best way to deal with anxiety is to focus on your senses. Do something physical like dancing, listen to music, rub a piece of velvet or silk fabric, inhale a pleasurable smell such lavender or other aromatherapy oils. There is actual science behind the phrase "stop and smell the roses." In addition to lavender and rose, other popular aromatherapy oils are cypress, eucalyptus, fennel, geranium, ginger, lemon, lemongrass, patchouli, peppermint, rosemary, and tea tree, among others.

Ways to Deal With Personal Stress

The first step in dealing with stress is to recognize the symptoms and closely monitor them. If there is a pattern of negative behavior, then begin to take action. The following activity can help you gain control of your stress.

> ## Activity: Let It Go!
>
> - Make a list of things that are causing you stress, worry, or anxiety and keeping you from being as effective as you would like to be.
> - Carefully review your list and identify those that you can control (or to some degree, influence). Put a checkmark or star next to those items.
> - Then "let the rest go"!

When you are feeling overwhelmed or becoming consumed with anxiety or worry, your mantra should be "Let it go!" In fact, I have a sign on my credenza next to my computer that says just that. It is a helpful reminder to practice what I teach.

Coping Strategies

There are three ways of dealing with stress. The first is to eliminate/reduce the stressor or change your response to it. The second is to use the coping resources available to you. The third is to acquire or develop new coping resources or strategies. Let's look at each of these more closely.

When trying to eliminate or reduce the stressor, it often comes down to two words: control and choices. As mentioned earlier, people become stressed when they perceive a loss of control. As noted in the "Let it go!" activity, we have more control than we think we do. Often it requires us to make choices, and those choices are based on our values, our preferences, and our circumstances. It is important to remember that although we may not like the choices available to us, we do have choices. Here is an example:

> During the same seminar on "Managing Priorities and Stress" for the Wall Street firm, I asked people to write down their biggest stressors and then share them with the group. Sam stated that his biggest stressor was his commute. He lived in the Pocono Mountains and commuted every day via bus to Lower Manhattan. That meant he had to get up at

3:30 AM to get ready for work and board the bus. The commute home sometimes was longer, and he often didn't arrive home until 9:00 PM. No wonder he was stressed!

I suggested that we explore his options. He could either move closer to work or find a job closer to home. He didn't see it that way. He liked living in the mountains, and the cost of living would be higher if he moved closer to New York. He liked his job and didn't want to find something closer to home. To him, he had no choice but to continue that daily grind. He refused to accept that he had made a choice. He had chosen to maintain his grueling and stress-producing lifestyle.

Whether you realize it or not, you have many coping resources at your disposal. Some are health-related as described in Chapter 5, "Get Physical." These include nutrition, exercise, and sleep, to name a few. Other coping resources such as family, friends, and community were addressed in Chapter 3, "Stay Connected." The amount of closeness we feel with others greatly affects our ability to cope with stress. As we discovered during the pandemic lockdown, closeness is essential to our psychological, emotional, spiritual, and even physical well-being. Perhaps the most important relationship you have is with yourself. That is why, self-care is so important.

Another coping resource is flexibility. Flexibility is essential not only in managing stress but also in helping us remain relevant. How often have you heard someone say (or maybe have said it yourself), "I can't change"? My response to that comment is "can't or won't"? As human beings, we have the ability to change, and the willingness to change will help us remain relevant. Let's look at some actions you can take to gain and maintain control of your circumstances. Self-management is key. One effective self-management technique is delegation. Learn to delegate both at home and at work. Of course, if you live alone that becomes more problematic; however, you can draw on the resources at your disposal. Granted, you may have to pay for services that will ease your burden, but it is still a form of delegation.

Stress Management Techniques

Begin practicing stress-reduction techniques. These include exercise, massage therapy, meditation, and relaxation. Do whatever works for you.

Deep Breathing

One effective technique that you can practice anywhere at any time is deep breathing. You can sit, stand, or lie down. The key is to breathe in deeply from your diaphragm and through your nose, then exhale slowly through your mouth. Repeating this a dozen or so times will help you get control.

Muscle Relaxation

You might also try muscle relaxation. It is best to lie down for this, but you can also do it in a sitting position. The effect is further enhanced by listening to specific recordings in which a professional takes you through the process. In a nutshell, muscle relaxation involves tightening and releasing the muscles in your body, one area or body part at a time, starting with your feet and moving upward.

Visualization

Visualization is also helpful. Get comfortable and begin visualizing a place where you would like to be. It could be the ocean, a babbling brook, or a mountain lake. Close your eyes and picture your quiet place, focusing on how pleasant it is and how relaxed you are.

Activity: Visualization Exercise

1. Picture your quiet place in as much detail as possible. Think about the following:
   - What are you wearing?   What time of day is it?
   - What do you see?   What time of year is it?
   - What do you hear?   Where are you sitting?
   - What do you smell?   What do you feel?

2. Turn on a piece of recorded music that relaxes you. It could be classical or environmental music or even just environmental sounds such as a babbling brook or ocean waves breaking on the shore.

3. Place yourself in a comfortable spot, loosen your belt, and remove your shoes if you like.

4. Close your eyes and breathe slowly in and out. Focus on breathing deeply from your diaphragm. Inhale slowly and deeply for four seconds, counting 1, 2, 3, 4 in your head. Then exhale slowly, mentally counting four seconds. Picture yourself in your special place as you concentrate on breathing in and out.

5. As you continue breathing deeply, listening to the relaxing soothing sounds, and picturing yourself in your special place, focus your attention on your muscle groups. Begin by tensing the muscles in your feet, holding the tension, and then relaxing the muscles. Notice the difference between the tense and relaxed states. Next, tense and then relax your leg muscles, and continue this process with every muscle group, moving up through the body to the face, neck, and head.

6. Continue breathing deeply. As you breathe in, mentally say to yourself, "I am…" And as you breathe out, say to yourself, "…relaxed." Continue breathing in and out and mentally reciting this mantra for the next ten minutes.

7. When you are finished with your deep-breathing and progressive muscle relaxation exercises, open your eyes and return to your immediate surroundings feeling relaxed and refreshed.

Self-Management

You may need to take a time management course or get help from your manager in setting priorities. Try to reshape your job. Learn new skills. Build a support system both inside and outside your workplace. Be kind to yourself. Practice positive self-talk and schedule time for yourself. Most of all, learn to have fun.

In addition to taking action on those over which you have some control or influence, identify and learn to accept those things you cannot do anything about. Then let it go! Realize that you do have choices and options. You can choose to take control or be controlled. If you choose to take control, you have many tools and resources available to help you experience the harmony you seek.

In our quest for harmony, we cannot ignore the more abstract, nebulous, and often nuanced elements of our being. The psychological, spiritual, and emotional aspects of our lives are intertwined, and if one is not functioning properly, the other two will suffer as well.

Self-Care

The Self-Care Forum's definition of self-care is "the actions that individuals take for themselves on behalf of and with others to develop, protect, maintain, and improve their health, wellbeing, or wellness." In short, it is about taking conscious actions to promote your physical, mental, and emotional health. Self-care takes many forms. Although we addressed physical health in Chapter 5, "Get Physical" and mental health in Chapter 1, "Stay Sharp," they bear repeating as crucial elements of self-care. Some people regard self-care as selfish and self-centered. There is a reason the flight attendant instructs passengers to put on their oxygen masks before attending to others. You cannot help anyone, not even yourself, if you don't take care of yourself first. As writer and poet Audre Lorde once stated, "Self-care is not self-indulgence; it is self-preservation."

At some point in our lives, we have all struggled with self-doubt and feelings of inadequacy. As we age, we may begin to feel that we are no longer as valuable as we once were. Sometimes, self-reflection can help bolster our self-esteem.

Self-Reflection

- Write down three things you appreciate about yourself.
- Ask a trusted friend to tell you what strengths they see in you.

You will be amazed at how much better you feel about yourself after taking these two actions.

Say "No"

One overlooked self-care practice is saying *no*. A major contributing factor to our stress is other people who make demands on our time. Although we may not be able to eliminate them, we can manage them by learning to say *no*. How often have you found yourself overwhelmed and overcommitted because you didn't say *no*? Notice I said *didn't*, not *couldn't*. In so many situations, we chose not to say *no* for a variety of reasons and then suffered the consequences by feeling overwhelmed, resentful, or unappreciated. We should be able to say *no* to activities that don't add value to our lives. As Roy Blauss, author of inspirational messages, puts it, "We should cultivate the ability to say no to activities for which we have no time, no talent and for which we have no real interest or real concern. If we learn to say no to many things, then we will be able to say yes to the things that matter most."

To cultivate that ability, begin by determining the underlying reason preventing you from saying *no*. Here are a few likely culprits:

- Feel obligated
- Don't want to hurt the other person's feelings
- Afraid people won't like you
- Prove you can *do it all*

Once you have identified the underlying cause, now it's time to revisit your values and your life wheel. Is saying *yes* congruent with what is important to you? Remember: your values, including the importance of relationships, should drive your choices and your behavior.

Should you choose to turn down the request, you will need to act while preserving the relationship with the person who made the request. I suggest you craft a template for your response to be delivered in person, over the telephone, or via e-mail. Please, no text messages!

- Begin by expressing appreciation to the person for thinking of you.
- Develop rapport by making a connection.

- Gracefully and tactfully turn down the request and your reason for doing so.
- Reaffirm the relationship and keep the door open.

Someone has asked you several times to get together for lunch or dinner, and you have put them off by offering excuses. You keep hoping the person will take the hint and stop asking. However, the person is tenacious. Rather than offer more excuses or bluntly telling the person you aren't interested in getting together, consider the following:

"Thanks for reaching out. It is so nice to hear from you. I imagine this past year has been as stressful for you as it has been for me. Given that I'm feeling a bit overwhelmed, I have decided to take a break from networking and not add anything more to my plate right now. That said, I would like to keep in touch. Let's plan on connecting in a few months once my schedule is less hectic. In fact, I'm going to put it on my calendar to contact you in three months and set a date for getting together. Does that work for you?"

Practice Planned Unavailability

Schedule time for yourself by practicing planned unavailability (PU). Look at your calendar—both personal and professional. I imagine it is chock full of meetings, medical appointments, volunteer activities, family obligations, and other commitments—dates and associated time frames. Don't get me wrong. These are all very important, especially if they are consistent with your values. I can also imagine that there is one thing noticeably absent on your busy schedule: time for yourself. What *time for yourself* means will vary from person to person.

Time Management

Sometimes we are so tightly scheduled that it is no wonder we are stressed and frazzled. If you find yourself running from one thing to another, it's time to stop and assess how you are spending your time and how realistic you are.

A Self-Assessment: Time Management

Instructions: For each of the following items, place a checkmark indicating if you practice that behavior or apply that technique.

	Yes	*No*	*Sometimes*

1. I have a written list of business goals.
2. I have a written list of personal goals.
3. I keep track of my progress toward accomplishing my goals.
4. I keep a master list of tasks I need to do daily.
5. I make a fresh new *to do* list each day.
6. I prioritize my various jobs and activities.
7. I estimate the time required for each activity on my daily *to do* list.
8. I break down large tasks into smaller ones to make sure they are accomplished.
9. I keep a record of how I spend my time.
10. I analyze how I am spending my time to improve my performance.
11. I develop a visible weekly plan that includes goals, priorities, and activities.
12. I schedule time for important tasks daily.
13. I work to minimize interruptions.
14. I group items such as paperwork, e-mails, return calls, and so on to handle several things effectively.
15. I keep a tickler file or some other system for tracking and follow-up.
16. I delegate as much as I can both at work and at home.
17. I do as much as I can to get things started even if I'm not in the mood.
18. I use effective techniques for saying *no* to overwhelming demands of my time.

	Yes	No	Sometimes
19. I allow time for unexpected things in my schedule.			
20. I regularly schedule quiet time (*Me Time*) in my daily plan.			

Look at the items you checked *No* or *Sometimes* and then decide if you would like to improve in that area. If so, develop an action plan to change or modify your behavior.

It is important to note that there is no such thing as time management. It's really self-management, that is, how we manage ourselves with respect to time. It is possible to influence, if not control, externally generated time problems. It is, however, much more difficult to identify and manage our internally generated time wasters.

I was coaching an executive vice president of a media company who was clearly feeling stressed and overwhelmed. It was affecting him both personally and professionally. He was proud of the fact that he had no down time and was able to cram so much into each day. When I looked at his calendar, it was obvious to me that he was the source of his distress. He was overscheduled! For example, he scheduled meetings back-to-back. That is a problem even if the meetings are in the same location, but frequently he would be scheduled for a meeting from 9:00 to 10:00 am and then another one from 10:00 to 11:00 in a building a mile away. Unless he had the ability to transport himself from one place to another in an instant, the timeframe was impossible. No wonder he was frazzled! The duress caused by this tightly packed schedule was further exacerbated because he had not scheduled one minute for himself—even on weekends. I suggested that he start making appointments with himself and set aside time on his calendar for "me time." I also convinced him to be more realistic in scheduling meetings and build in "fluff time" such as time for travel between locations, making allowances for unexpected occurrences such as meetings running over the allotted time, grabbing a cup of coffee, or taking a "bio break."

Your Psychological Well-Being

Psychological well-being is an important contributing factor to remaining relevant. Self-awareness, self-acceptance, and positive self-talk are just a few elements of psychological well-being. Consider some of the techniques you can practice to maintain a mentally healthy state.

Mindfulness

Mindfulness is a therapeutic technique that, simply put, means focusing on awareness of the present moment. It can help you explore spirituality by heightening your awareness of the present moment. It involves becoming acutely aware of and acknowledging our thoughts, feelings, and bodily sensations and then accepting them. We are often so focused on the future or obsessed with the past that we don't know how to be in the moment and relish it as an amazing gift. If you have any doubt, look around you when you are visiting a tourist spot or out to dinner. Notice that people are so busy taking *selfies* that they lose sight of the experience before them. How often have you noticed people at a restaurant who are more interested in taking pictures of the food on their plates instead of enjoying and savoring the tastes, aromas, and the artistry of the food presentation? Speaking of dining out, have you noticed how many people who are out with friends and family spend more time checking messages or texting than being engaged in conversation with their dining companions?

Mindfulness involves an acute awareness of the five senses: sight, sound, touch, smell, and taste. To gain a better understanding of their impact, try the following activity.

Activity: Sensory Awareness

Choose a food item or something that you would be able to experience all five senses as you ingest it.

- What does it look like? Really look at the color and texture.
- What does it smell like? Take a deep breath savoring the aroma as it enters your nose.

> • What does it feel like? Is it hot or cold, mild or spicy?
> What sensation do you experience?
> • What sound does it make as you eat it? Is it crunchy or
> does it roll effortlessly over your tongue?

Meditation

You might also try meditation. Meditation and mindfulness are often used interchangeably. While they are inter-related, they are indeed different. Meditation refers to a formal, seated practice. During meditation, you intentionally focus inward to increase awareness, concentration, and calmness. Meditation is a tool to develop mindfulness. You can practice mindfulness during formal meditation sessions.

Affirmations and Mantras

What are affirmations and do they really work? Affirmations are phrases that you repeat to yourself regularly that describe a desired outcome or how you want to be or see yourself. At first, affirmations may seem silly and even a waste of time. They are positive statements that help you reprogram your mind. Affirmations work on the subconscious and are designed to encourage an optimistic mindset. Studies show that repeated positive affirmations lead to positive thinking, and positive thinking leads to positive action and results. Start with something easy to remember. The Internet has no shortage of examples of affirmations. Two great resources for different types of affirmations are www.positivepsycholgy.com/daily-affirmations and www.prolificliving.com/100-positive-affirmations.

If you choose to create your own (highly recommended and preferred), follow this formula developed by noted motivational speaker and co-author of the *Chicken Soup for the Soul* series, Jack Canfield. For a more detailed explanation, visit Jack's "Daily Affirmations for Success" on his website (www.jackcanfield.com).

1. Start with "I am."
2. Use a present tense verb ending with "ing."
3. State it in the positive.

4. Keep it brief—no more than 15 words
5. Make it specific.
6. Include a word that conveys emotion.

Using his formula, I created two affirmations for myself:

"I am excited that I am walking across the stage at age 49 to accept my PhD." This is an affirmation I started at age 40 as I was considering enrolling in a doctorate program.

"I am delighted that I am sitting with a talk show host discussing my book." This affirmation is one that I have started repeating when I began work on this book.

Notice how nicely the affirmation fits with visualization. While reciting my affirmation, I visualize what I am wearing, the time of day, and what is around me. To be effective, you should repeat your affirmations three to five times a day.

You might also find mantras to be helpful. While mantras are similar to affirmations, they are not the same. In the context of its origin, a mantra is a sound or word repeated to aid in concentration used in accordance with meditation. In its popular usage, a mantra now includes a phrase or slogan repeated frequently to help promote positive thinking.

Examples:

I am successful

I am at peace.

My current personal mantra is "Let it go!"

Yoga

In Chapter 5, "Get Physical," we explored the physical benefits of yoga. Yet yoga has psychological, emotional, and spiritual benefits as well. There is a mind–body connection in the practice of yoga, resulting in less stress, improved self-esteem, and increased inner strength. According to Dr. Natalie Nevins, an osteopathic physician and yoga instructor in Hollywood, California, "Regular yoga practice creates mental clarity and calmness; increases body awareness; relieves chronic stress patterns; relaxes the mind; centers attention; and sharpens concentration."

Spirituality

What is spirituality? Spirituality is about seeking a connection with something bigger than ourselves and results in positive emotions. It may or may not involve formal religion. It brings meaning and purpose to your life and involves relationships, values, and life purpose. Spirituality also helps you to understand and connect with the universe, a sense of something bigger than ourselves—search for meaning in life. Religion and spirituality are not the same thing nor are they mutually exclusive. Spirituality is a much broader concept than religion and may incorporate elements of religion. Religion helps us determine right from wrong and what is true and false. It provides us with a moral compass and keeps us grounded while spirituality gives us meaning, connection, value.

Tips for Seeking Harmony

- Practice relaxation techniques such as meditation, yoga, deep breathing exercises, and muscle relaxation.
- Use visualization. Practice seeing yourself as succeeding in difficult or anxiety-producing situations.
- Practice good nutritional habits such as eating regular healthy meals, eliminating *junk food*, and eating five fruits and vegetables each day.
- Incorporate a regular exercise program into your daily/weekly schedule.
- Treat yourself to regular massage therapy sessions.
- Use effective time management techniques to increase effectiveness and productivity. Set and prioritize goals, make daily *to do* lists, set realistic deadlines, and get control of your e-mails.
- Delegate tasks and responsibilities both at home and at work.
- Overcome procrastination by creating deadlines and breaking down projects into manageable *chunks* and doing one thing at a time.

- Practice assertive skills at work and at home. Don't allow others (or yourself) to overburden you. Learn to say *no*.
- Establish a support network of family, friends, and other resources. Rely on others to help you *lighten your load*. Do not be afraid to ask for help and accept help when it is offered.

Take Action!

- Practice one stress management technique each day.
- Incorporate one new time management technique into your daily or weekly schedule.
- Create an affirmation for yourself and repeat it at least three times a day.

CHAPTER 7

Keep Up With Technology

Technology is best when it brings people together.
—Matt Mullanweg, Social Media Entrepreneur

"I hate technology!"
"Technology intimidates me."
"I'm too old to learn all this new technology."
"Things were a lot simpler before technology took over."
"Technology is not my friend."

Do any of these statements sound familiar to you? Have you said them or at least thought them? If so, you are a technophobe, and you are not alone. Like it or not, technology is a major part of our professional and personal lives. In today's business environment, no one can deny the importance of technology. You don't have to master technology to become tech savvy, but you can't shy away from it either if you want to be perceived as relevant.

Reasons Older People Shy Away From Technology

A 2020 survey of adults over age 60 conducted by Candoo Tech (www .candootech.com) shows that 53 percent of older adults fear learning a new tech device is more frightening than hearing a strange noise at night, going to the dentist, and going to the doctor combined. While this informal poll did not differentiate among people who are no longer working, have never worked, or are still engaged in their careers, it underscores how stressful and challenging technology can be for those who are older. Furthermore, articles addressing people who shy away from technology referred to the population as *elderly, seniors,* or *geriatric.* One such article was entitled "Geriatric Technophobia" and discussed the population as though anyone over 65 had *checked out* of the workforce. Although all the studies and articles I reviewed focused on a general population of people over 65, the point is that many older adults (working or not) are afraid of technology. Why?

Fear

- Fear of the unknown or uncertainty based on the lack of information or knowledge.
- Fear of failure, making a mistake, or breaking the computer.
- Fear of feeling inadequate. What comes as natural to those who are younger than we are, is a challenge for many in the 65+ category. We didn't grow up with technology, so we have to learn new skills.
- Fear of being vulnerable—safety and privacy issues, especially when we hear about organizations and individuals being hacked and information stolen.

Lack of Motivation

- Not interested in investing the time and effort. As we age, it does take more time to learn new things; however, the will to and practice of learning something new can aid brain functioning.
- The number of devices and applications can be overwhelming.
- Do not see the benefits or need.

To overcome the fears and lack of motivation, the first place to start is to examine the benefits of technology as they apply to your business or career.

Benefits of Technology for Your Business or Career

In conducting research for this chapter, all the articles citing benefits to the over-65 population primarily focus on older adults wanting to stay connected with their children and grandchildren. While this is important to your personal life, I want to address how keeping up with technology can help you remain relevant in your professional life as well.

- Access information about anything
- Enables you to keep up with trends
- Follow thought leaders and key influencers
- Help people retain their cognitive skills as they age

Techie Terminology

Most likely, if you are still actively engaged in your career, you are familiar with the technology associated with your business. If so, you can skip this section. However, we cannot make assumptions. Much to my surprise, I discovered that many professionals prior to the pandemic had never heard of Zoom. To this day, many of those folks wish they hadn't. Even if you are confident in your knowledge of technology terminology, you may want to revisit key terms to make sure you understand them.

Activity: Terms and Definitions

Match the term in the first column with the definition in the second column.

1. Bandwidth	a. Live video-based meeting between people in different locations
2. Browser	b. Small text sent by a website you have visited
3. Application	c. Permanent storage of data
4. Virus, Spyware, Trojan, Malware	d. Unsolicited e-mail message sent out in bulk

5. Videoconferencing	e. A program enabling people to use the computer for a specific task or function
6. Cloud	f. A piece of computer software or hardware that blocks data from flowing through
7. Memory	g. Strings of letters and numbers that have to be typed in on some web pages to block spam
8. Disk Space	h. Temporary storage used by a computer when computer is on
9. Phishing	i. Piece of software that can copy itself and attach itself to another program generally for malicious intent
10. Cookie	j. A program used to look at pages on the web
11. Firewall	k. Refers to how quickly data travels along a connection
12. Spam	l. Storing and accessing data and programs over the Internet
13. CAPTCHA	m. Fraudulent practice of sending e-mails for the purpose of gaining personal or confidential information

Mastering the Basic Tools

Review the following Google and Microsoft products and note which ones you use. Perhaps you are not even aware of the plethora of products that can help you become more effective, efficient, and relevant.

Google Products for Business

Search engine Google should be your *go to* place for information on anything! Whatever you want to know, Google can find it for you. In addition to being a powerful source for accessing data, Google has many products that can help you maximize your resources and productivity. Those that are highly recommended, especially for smaller businesses, include Calendar, Blogger, AdSense, Analytics, Google Meet, Google Marketing Platform, Surveys, and Google Workplace. For entrepreneurs, sole proprietors, professional services providers, Google Chrome has an abundance of tools to manage your business:

- E-mail (of course)
- Contacts (customer relationship management system)
- Docs (equivalent to Word)
- Sheets (equivalent to PowerPoint)
- Translate (if you deal with customers/clients for whom English is a second language)

Microsoft

Microsoft 365 is a productivity toolkit. Within this office suite are products that you are probably already using, but are you using them as effectively as you could? Are you using all of them? Do you know what they are? Office 365 includes Word, PowerPoint, Excel, One Note, Outlook, Publisher, and Teams.

Must-Have Social Media for Business

Social media presence and involvement are essential in today's business world. Most people think of social media in terms of marketing, and you should too if you are marketing your business or yourself. If that is the case, I suggest you do a *deep dive* into each to determine how you can use them to generate leads and promote your products and services. Your proficiency and comfort level with social media can go a long way in creating the perception of being relevant. Participating in social media goes beyond marketing and lead generation. Having a social media presence can contribute greatly to helping you remain relevant.

Benefits of Social Media Presence

- Access timely topics by listening to podcasts and watching videos.

- Stay connected with customers/clients. Keeps you fresh in their minds by posting articles, stories, pictures, and showcasing your efforts with social responsibility and sustainability.
- Keep on top of what your competitors are doing.
- Establish you as a thought leader.
- Engage your customers through messaging and texts.
- Greater exposure.
- Gain greater insight into your clients' concerns, wants, and needs.
- Help you appeal to younger, social-savvy customers.

Social media requires a significant time investment. To use social media effectively, you need to log into your account(s) at least once a day. If spending time learning and using social media is not where you want to focus your time and energy, then outsource. Again, look to younger members of your family, friends, neighbors for help. Colleges and universities are also good sources of *cheap labor*. In fact, interns may even be free.

Let's look at the most important social media platforms:

LinkedIn

Widely considered the benchmark for professional networking social media platforms, LinkedIn can give you and your company exposure you cannot get elsewhere. It gives you the opportunity to *see and be seen* by posting articles and responding to others' posts. Remember: it is not just who you know but who knows you. It is also useful as a research tool for information about other people and organizations and helps you remain competitive.

LinkedIn Groups

By joining LinkedIn Groups, you can stay on top of trends in your business or industry. It allows you to participate in discussion forums on specific business-focused topics. You become engaged in *gives* and *gets*. Within these forums, you can ask meaningful questions and give interesting answers to others. Through these engagements, you demonstrate your credibility and showcase your expertise. You start to be regarded as an influencer and a thought leader, indicators of being relevant. Within these groups, you can share quality content specific to your industry and position yourself as an expert or an authority.

LinkedIn Learning

LinkedIn Learning is a learning platform that you can use in two ways. First, you can learn new skills or acquire information on topics of interest to you. Unlike YouTube, there is a monthly fee, but the quality is more professional. Second, you can present courses you have developed. This is a great way to showcase your relevance in addition to connecting with people.

LinkedIn Events

LinkedIn Events is a networking and learning hub offering events in any industry. It enables you to connect with and learn from your peers. Whether you are a participant or an event host, your attendance and participation in these events helps you remain relevant.

LinkedIn Publishing

LinkedIn Publishing affords you the opportunity to publish original content. By sharing your thoughts and expertise, you add to your credibility and establish yourself as a thought leader.

In addition to helping you remain relevant, LinkedIn is a great networking resource for staying connected with colleagues and clients (as discussed in Chapter 3, "Stay Connected") while in your present position. Furthermore, these connections can prove to be invaluable if you decide to switch careers.

Instagram and Facebook for Business

Facebook and Instagram serve a different purpose from LinkedIn. Text-based and informational, Facebook is the gold standard when it comes to social media marketing. In addition to traditional marketing, it gives you the opportunity to enhance your brand awareness and drive website traffic. You may already be familiar with Facebook for personal use, but you can create a business page as well.

Instagram does not readily come to mind as applicable to business, but depending on your type of business, you may want to consider it as a supplement to Facebook. Keep in mind that Instagram is strictly image/video based and is used to engage the audience. For that reason, realtors find it particularly helpful.

Here is a great resource for how to choose the most suitable social media platform for your business: https://seopressor.com/blog/how-to-choose-social-media-for-business.

Websites

An up-to-date website is essential for today's business or businessperson who is not employed by someone else. A website lets people know who you are; what you do; how you do business; your products and services; your credentials; client testimonials. It is important to incorporate video, if you can. In addition to increasing client activity and interest, it demonstrates that you are in tune with what appeals to today's consumer. Be sure to hire a website designer/developer who is knowledgeable about current design trends.

Blogs

As a professional, you may already read blogs and you may even write one yourself. But for those of you who do not, consider blogging. A blog is such an effortless way to demonstrate that you are relevant. For those of you who may not be familiar with blogs, quite simply a blog is a type of website that focuses on written content. Because the information is presented from a personal perspective, it enables you really shine and display your knowledge and expertise. It includes a *comments* section that facilitates engagement and interaction with your readers. Blogging is inexpensive (can be free) and can be set up in a short time.

Why blog?

- Gets you and your business more exposure
- Establishes you as an expert and thought leader
- Generates passive income by selling your products and services and selling advertising space

Podcasts and YouTube Channels

Both Podcasts and YouTube are great vehicles to highlight your talents and prove your relevance. Just by the fact that you are engaging in one or both these media, you are demonstrating that you do add value. Think about your vast knowledge based on your years of experience. There is no doubt that you would have plenty to share with people.

YouTube

YouTube is a free video-streaming platform designed to share content. On your YouTube channel, you can produce lectures, demonstrations, training programs, and other educational and informational programs. The programs can range from short *how-to's* of a few minutes to longer seminars that could last an hour or more. Although your primary purpose for having a YouTube channel is to promote your business and/or yourself, you can also use it to generate income through various revenue streams such as selling your products or services, licensing your content, or affiliate marketing, among others.

Podcasts

Whereas YouTube is visual, a podcast is audio only, much like talk radio. This is a major benefit for those of us over 60. Because people cannot see us, they cannot make a judgment about our age or appearance. Yes, they may be able to hear aging in your voice, but if you keep your voice rich and strong as discussed in Chapter 5, "Get Physical," it will not be a problem.

Podcasts are easy to set up and are very convenient for people to access. Using your smartphone, you can listen to a podcast from about anywhere at any time—commuting, working out, doing chores, running errands, waiting for appointments.

When trying to decide which to use, Podcast or YouTube, consider the following:

- Initial investment cost
- Ongoing costs
- Ease of setup
- Time commitment
- Ease of production
- Ease of use/accessibility for audience

Teleconferencing

As a result of the pandemic, many of us were forced into teleconferencing. Some people welcomed it, but a vast number of people were fearful and resistant. The most popular teleconferencing software include Zoom, WebEx by Cisco, Google Meet, Microsoft Teams, GoToMeetings, and Skype for Business. Which one you use is going to be dictated by the organization you work for or your client's preference. On the other hand, if you oversee selecting which application to use, determine the criteria that are most important to you, then do your research to select the platform that meets your needs. Here are some criteria to consider:

Selection Criteria

- Cost
- Quality of video
- Type of meeting(s)
- Number of meetings
- Ease of use
- Number of participants
- Features/capabilities
  - Recording
  - Chat

- º Breakout rooms
- º Screen sharing
- º Polling
- Customer support

Like it or not, studies show that teleconferencing is here to stay. With that in mind, we need to master the art of virtual delivery by adhering to a few basic practices that will enable you to present yourself as professional, polished, and relevant.

Guidelines for Virtual Presentations

- Stand up (if possible).
- Use a professional, clutter-free background. Observe the backgrounds people on television use when they are presenting or being interviewed in their homes.
- Pay attention to lighting. Have a good front light. Position yourself so that you are facing a light source such as a window or lamp.
- Look directly into the computer's camera, and experiment with the height of your computer so that viewers are not looking up your nostrils.
- Get close to the screen so that it frames your head, neck, and shoulders.
- Be energetic and animated.
- Engage participants by asking questions and having them respond via chat or comment by unmuting themselves.
- Use interesting slides and visuals that are uncluttered and easy to read.
- Know the technology.
- If you are presenting in a formal setting, particularly if there are a lot of participants, ask someone else to help by monitoring the chats and dealing with breakout rooms.

Guidelines for Participants

- Put yourself on mute unless you have something to say.

- Position yourself so that light is in front of you.
- Keep your background clutter-free. Not only is it distracting, it also looks unprofessional.
- Avoid distracting habits.
- Do not eat while on a conference call.
- If you need to get up and leave the area, turn off your video until you return.
- Be engaged. Although it is tempting to multitask, resist doing so. People can tell.
- Make your location inaccessible to children and pets.
- Dress professionally, even if it is a casual environment.

How to Overcome Fear of Technology

Change Your Mindset

Identify the basis of your fear. Instead of resisting technology, embrace it and make it your friend. Think about the benefits as noted earlier. As self-taught, over 65, technology expert Paul Dougherty, a sales associate with Berkshire Hathaway Home Services in Glenside, Pennsylvania, puts it, "If people knew how much easier technology can make their lives, they would not be so afraid to use it."

Explore the Websites

Go to the websites of the applications and play around. Don't be afraid to click on the sidebars and see where they take you. It is amazing what you can learn just by exploring the websites.

Invest the Time

Take the time to learn the technology. That means you need to be doing something every day to enhance your knowledge of and proficiency in some aspect of technology.

Research

Here is where Google can really help. If you do not know how to do something, go to Google or YouTube.

Take Classes

Enroll in free online courses to learn how to use various applications such as Excel. You can also search for tutorials and YouTube videos. If your organization offers courses, be sure to take advantage of them. Not only will you learn how to use the technology, but you will also be demonstrating that you are not afraid to learn something new, and you are interested in being on the cutting edge.

Ask Questions

Although there are many social media platforms (such as TikTok) and instant messaging applications (such as Snapchat), you will never use, you should at least know what they are so that you are not perceived as a dinosaur. Ask your children or grandchildren to educate you on the latest trends in technology.

For help with platforms and applications specific to your organization, reach out to the technology experts/IT department to guide you. They are there to help.

Engage Outside Resources

If you are a small business owner, sole proprietor, or professional services provider, you may not have the time or inclination to keep up with technology. If that is the case, hire a contractor to help you. If cost is a factor, contact your local colleges and universities for interns.

Answers to Techie Terms and Definitions
1-k;2-j;3-e;4-i;5-a;6-l;7-h;8-c;9-m;10-b;11-f;12-d;13-g

Take Action!

- Join one or two LinkedIn groups.
- Create or update your website.
- Start a blog and/or podcast.
- Take a course to increase your knowledge of some aspect of technology.

CHAPTER 8

Reinvent Yourself

Life isn't about finding yourself. Life is about creating yourself.
—George Bernard Shaw, Irish Playwright

This final chapter is for those who want to be actively engaged in the work world but who may want to experience it differently. Either by choice or necessity, perhaps you want to start a new business or change careers. You may also choose to retire but not completely. According to a survey by the Employee Benefit Research Institute, "79 percent of U.S. workers expect to supplement their retirement by working for pay." You have a great opportunity to leverage years of experience, knowledge, and expertise to succeed in the next phase of your life, no matter what your age.

Starting a New Career

As mentioned in the Introduction, many famous people who accomplished amazing things did so well past the traditional retirement age. Several well-known people became successful after they switched careers later in life:

- Harland Sanders became the fried chicken mogul at 65 after having held various jobs before officially retiring and receiving a social security check.
- Anna Mary Robertson Moses (Grandma Moses) was 76 when she painted her first canvas and continued to paint for another 25 years.
- Laura Ingalls Wilder, author of the *Little House on the Prairie* series, who was a teacher prior to getting married, and later a poultry farmer didn't write her first novel until she was 65.

In addition to these notables, there are many people who started new careers later in life. Although they are lesser known, they are no less noteworthy. There are many ways to reinvent yourself. Some are intentional; others, accidental. Some are driven by desire; others out of necessity. Some changes are related to people's current careers; others chose to do something totally different.

Accidental Career Changes

Birtan Collier started a new career when her husband of 30 years died in 2013. Ralph Collier was a well-known voice in radio in the Philadelphia area, who interviewed celebrities and newsworthy figures. Birtan, a former banker and political adviser, stepped up to the microphone to keep the show going, and she continues to interview authors and noteworthy people even today. Not only is she a self-proclaimed news junkie, she remains relevant by practicing self-care, keeping herself physically and mentally healthy. Birtan reads about what is happening in technology and uses her natural curiosity to continue to learn. She believes in trying to find something positive even in our darkest hours. She advises people to "set goals, take the initiative, create opportunities, and not leave things to chance."

Evolutional Career Paths

Many people in the latter part of their careers look back and ask themselves, "How did I get here?" They are products of an unintended career path that just somehow evolved over time. As part of their journeys, they acquired valuable skills through experience that have served them well and resulted in their success.

Paul Dougherty's new career in real estate at age 64 evolved from his business as a home painting contractor. It seemed like a natural extension of what he had been doing for many years. Always curious about technology, Paul became a self-taught computer techie and is the tech specialist in his real estate office.

Over her lengthy career in publication, Vilma Barr has worn many hats. She began her career as a contributing writer for consumer publications, and 55 years later, she is still writing and communicating ideas about the physical world. Along the way, Vilma was the head of public relations for a civil engineering firm, edited books for McGraw-Hill, and co-authored several books on the side. Today, she is a publishing consultant to authors of nonfiction books, assisting "authors in the development of their creative writing skills and placement of their books with an internationally distributed publisher."

Intentional Career Changes

Rosemary Browne had a long and successful career as a clinical operations manager for two large health care systems. After officially leaving the workforce at age 65, she spent the next six months focused on her volunteer work. She has a passion for animals and has been an active volunteer for 11 years at Providence Animal Center, where she is involved in the dog foster program. Other animal-related volunteer activities include being a home visitor for Delaware Valley Golden Retriever Rescue and helping disabled riders at a riding academy. She has volunteered at the Citizen Corps of Delaware County (Pennsylvania) and does food pantry work along with her husband Rick. Although she felt relevant through her volunteer work, she needed more and decided she wanted to do something that again would provide a paycheck even though she didn't need the money. As she said, "There is something about getting a paycheck that makes you feel valued." A friend suggested substitute teaching, which she has been doing for the past few years. Although she teaches only three or four days a week, she is in such demand, she could do it full time. She loves interacting with the students and staff. Not only does she feel valued and appreciated, but she also remains relevant by engaging with the students, knowing what they read, what they watch on television, and what they want. Teaching has required her to learn new skills and get out of her comfort zone.

At the height of his career, Dr. Robert Brookman transitioned from pulmonary medicine/critical care medicine to the practice of anti-aging, regenerative, and functional medicine. Changes in the health care system and burnout prompted Dr. Brookman to explore other avenues within the medical profession. With some skepticism, he attended his first conference on anti-aging and spent the next two years reading, attending conferences, and getting certified in the practice of anti-aging medicine. His holistic approach to health is summarized by this Alex Huxley quotation: "I want my patients to die as young as they can as late as they can." Although he never left the medical profession, Dr. Brookman intentionally made a change from practicing traditional medicine to promoting the total well-being of his patients.

Approach to Reinventing Yourself

Reinventing yourself does not just happen. It is an intentional process that involves many of the same initiatives you used when you first started your career many years ago.

Begin With a Positive Mindset

"I'm too old to start over."
"You can't teach an old dog new tricks."
"My time has passed."

Are you guilty of saying or thinking any of the aforementioned? Get them out of your head—now! You are never too old to learn something new. Eliminate the limiting beliefs and negative self-talk, and replace them with positive thoughts. If you have not already, now would be a good time to start incorporating the positive affirmations addressed in Chapter 6, "Seek Harmony" into your daily life.

Also eliminate the *wouldas, couldas,* and *shouldas* that may be plaguing you. All three focus on the past and imply failure. Instead, focus on the future with "I will…" or "I am going to…." There are no *do-overs* in life; therefore, the backward-focused thoughts are irrelevant. We cannot change the past, but we can learn from it and move on. Age may be a number, but it does not have to be a state of mind.

Follow Your Passion

Pursue your passion, and you will find success. Each one of us must define success for ourselves—not benchmark against someone else or some ideal image of what success looks like or feels like. Passion, that intense enthusiasm for something, makes you feel alive and gives you purpose. Several of the people I interviewed said that to remain relevant, you must have a sense of purpose. It's what makes you want to get up in the morning. As the late Katherine Graham, formerly publisher of the *Washington Post*, once said, "To love what you do and feel that it matters—how could anything be more fun?"

For example, animal welfare is one of my passions. Through a networking contact, I was approached by the board president of Providence Animal Center, Jo-Ann Zoll, who became aware of my interest and suggested that I would be well-suited volunteering in fundraising/development. Although animal welfare is my passion, raising money is not. Besides, I'm not good at it. In addition to animals, my other passion is developing people. After giving it a lot of thought, I said to her, "I don't scoop poop and I don't ask people for money. What I will do is offer my consulting and training services to train the staff in leadership, team building, and goal setting. My contribution is that I would be helping the people who help the animals and take care of them."

Melissa Davey

Melissa Davey knows about following your passion. At age 65, she decided to live her dream of becoming a film producer, launching her first documentary film, *The Beyond Sixty Project*. The film focuses on 10 women over 60 who are determined to remain relevant. These professional women range in age from their 60s to mid-80s who come from different parts of the country and different backgrounds. She was drawn to this project by her burning desire to hear stories about ordinary women who have done and continue to do amazing things despite ageism and the negativity toward older women in advertising and the media. Melissa is an example of someone who continues to overcome the arbitrary division and the either-or mindset of working versus being retired.

When she decided to leave her job as a corporate executive to pursue her new career, people around her, including family and friends, could not understand that she was not retiring. In people's minds, when you no longer have a title or are no longer receiving a paycheck, then your work life is over. Melissa, as well as the women in the film, are truly inspiring.

Acknowledging that society makes assumptions and perceptions about age, and that those judgments must be broken down for us to remain relevant, she asserts that people need to take responsibility for remaining relevant. As she puts it, "That means continuing to grow and be engaged with the rest of the world. You need to be curious as to how the world works, be open-minded, challenge yourself, and accept change. It's important to surround yourself with different people and especially younger folks." Like many others I spoke with, Melissa mentioned the importance of having a purpose.

Beyond Sixty was released on April 6, 2021, and is available on demand and through most streaming channels.

Activity: Fired Up!

To further explore and define your passion, answer the following questions:

- What gets you excited or energizes you?
- What makes you want to get up in the morning?
- What would you like to do even if you didn't get paid to do it?

Reinvention Process

The path ahead of you is much shorter than the path behind you. Thus, you have no time to waste. Just as you did at the beginning of your career, you need to follow a process by addressing the following questions:

Where am I now?
Where do I want to go?
How do I get there?

Take Personal Stock: Where Am I Now?

At this point in your life, you are acutely aware of your likes and dislikes, personal characteristics, skills, accomplishments, strengths and weaknesses, and interests. Now it's time to go deeper as you take a personal inventory. One helpful tool to use in self-assessment is to reflect on your personal values you completed in Chapter 6, "Seek Harmony."

Although your priorities may change based on life circumstances, your basic values do not. For example, *Physical and Mental Health* may always have been something you valued, but that category may now have a higher priority due to your current health situation or that of a family member.

This is also a good time to revisit your Life Wheel in Chapter 6, "Seek Harmony." If, for example, you ranked *Mental and Physical Health* high on your values assessment, but the *pie slice* on your Real Wheel is small in comparison to that of your Ideal Wheel, you are not congruent. Furthermore, you are probably stressed because your behavior does not support what you say is important to you.

Personal Inventory

As you consider what you want to do with the rest of your work life, in addition to completing the *What Do I Value?* assessment and the *Life Wheel* activity, it can be helpful to make a list of your personal critical success factors. This individual inventory serves as a basis for your reinvention and provides intrinsic reward as you reflect with pride and satisfaction on your stellar career.

- Skills
- Accomplishments
- Personal traits
- Talents
- Expertise

Clarify Your Vision: Where Do I Want to Go?

A personal vision is a general statement of your future as you would like it to be. *Just as you had a personal vision when you started your career, you need one for your new career.* In case you have forgotten how to create a personal vision, you can start by addressing the following questions:

- Where do you see yourself in two years? Five years?
- What are you doing?
- Where are you physically located?
- Who is around you?

Create a Vision Board

An effective tool to help you with your personal reinvention is a vision board. A vision board goes deeper than the affirmations and visualizations discussed in Chapter 6, "Seek Harmony." A vision board is a visual representation of your personal vision and goals. It is a collage of images, objects, statements, or words that represent the future you want to create.

Purpose/Benefits of a Vision Board

The Law of Attraction, first introduced in the early 19th century, is the theory behind the vision board. According to the theory, we can attract whatever we are focusing on. Studies support that the visual representation of our goals has a powerful impact on our subconscious mind. Over time, the visual representations begin to manifest and become a reality.

How to Make a Vision Board

1. Decide on a theme or what you want it to represent.
2. Begin collecting items, words, photos, cartoons, quotations, magazine clippings, stickers that relate to your theme.
3. Choose a board for your base. It can be cork, magnetic whiteboard, poster board, or some other medium. You may also choose to create it digitally.
4. Determine the size of the board and where you want to display it.
5. Start arranging and rearranging the items you assembled. Once you have them in place, secure them with push pins, glue, tape, or magnets.
6. Leave some space open to add other items that inspire you.
7. Place your vision board where you can see it regularly.
8. Create more than one vision board if you are visualizing and setting goals for different areas of your life.

How to Use Your Vision Board

A great way to achieve your goals is to keep them at the top of your mind. Put it in a prominent location where you can see it every day. Get into the habit of starting or ending each day looking at your vision board and reflecting on what you have done to realize the vision or goals represented.

If you would like more ideas for creating a vision board, a great free resource is Jack Canfield's "21 Ways to Make Your Vision Board More Powerful." (www.jackcanfield.com/blog/how-to-create-an-empowering-vision-board)

I remember attending a professional conference early in my career as a consultant. My two colleagues and I were on our way back to the hotel after attending morning sessions and visiting hundreds of vendors at the Expo in the afternoon. Many of the booths showcased authors who spoke about their published books and conducted book signings. I told my colleagues that I had a vision of my presenting to an audience of hundreds and then signing my published books at the Expo. They laughed and politely said, "Sure, Karen." My vision became a reality a few years later.

Branding Elements

At the core of reinventing yourself is the process of personal branding. Similar to a company's brand, a personal brand is a conscious and intentional effort to influence people's perception of us. It is never too late to create a new personal brand or elevate your existing one. By the mere fact that you are where you are in your career and have achieved success, you already have a brand. As Jeff Bezos puts it, "Your brand is what people say about you when you're not in the room." Do you know what people say about you? How do people perceive you? Are you perceived the way you want to be perceived? To help you clearly define your brand, ask yourself the following questions:

- What do I believe in?
- What do I value?
- What words would people use to describe me?
- What words would I use to describe myself?

- What makes me different from others with similar backgrounds?
- What do I do well?
- What makes people want to be around me?

You can discover the answers to many of these questions by completing the self-assessments, checklists, and activities presented throughout *Remaining Relevant.* If you have, go back and review them to gain additional personal insight. If you haven't, I encourage you to do so.

Rebranding Example

Dr. Gayle Carson is the quintessential role model for self-reinvention. Up until her death in August 2021 at age 83, the five-time breast cancer survivor was still going strong hosting 12 radio shows a month and appearing as a guest on podcasts, TV shows, and radio. Gayle's schedule was amazing. Like the Energizer Bunny, she kept going and going until the very end. Every day she would strap on her prosthesis, don her wig, and out the door she went. She shared with me that she had reinvented herself seven times. She started her career in broadcasting, then transitioned to become the owner of seven career schools followed by owning and running a modeling agency. She was also a spokesperson for Clairol, traveling the country interviewing women and giving them complete makeovers. Along the way, she earned her doctorate and became an international author and speaker on business. A few years ago, Gayle rebranded herself as the "Spunky Old Broad," "S.O.B." for short. Her target audience was women over 50, offering online programs and person-to-person or group coaching to help them succeed in their careers.

Set Goals

It is time to dust off those goal-setting skills you mastered years ago. Just as was the case when you started your career, you need to set goals as you launch a new one. Although your timeline is shorter than at the beginning of your career, goal setting is even more important because you have a shorter time to accomplish what you want.

The importance of goal setting cannot be overlooked. Do you remember when Alice asks the Cheshire Cat for help in choosing the right road in *Alice in Wonderland* by Lewis Carroll? The Cheshire Cat asked Alice, "Where are you going?" Alice replied, "I don't know." "Well," said the Cheshire Cat, "Then it doesn't matter which road you take."

To recap, here are the goal-setting criteria:

Specific—What exactly do you want to achieve?
Measurable—How are you going to quantify your progress?
Attainable—Can it be done, and do you have the ability to do it?
Relevant—Is the goal in harmony with your values and life purpose?
Timebound—When is the goal to be achieved?

As I mentioned in Chapter 1, "Stay Sharp," I set a goal to earn my PhD by the time I turned 50. At the same time, I added two more goals. I planned to have my CSP (Certified Speaking Professional, an earned designation from the National Speakers Association) and publish my first book. I'm proud to say that I met all three a year early.

Action Plan/Execution: How Do I Get There?

As the French writer, Antoine de Saint Exupéry, once wrote, "A goal without a plan is just a wish." Once you have your goal(s), it is imperative that you map out a plan with specific steps and timelines. This is where your project management skills come into play. Now *you* are the project.

Resilience

At this point in your life, you have undoubtedly demonstrated a great deal of resilience, both personally and professionally. As you move on to the next chapter in your life, you will need to continue to practice it. The ability to bounce back is critical to success. People can learn a lot from the Weeble, the roly-poly children's toy created in 1971 by Hasbro.

When the egg-shaped toy is tapped or knocked over, it causes the weight located at the bottom to be lifted off the ground. Once released, gravity brings the toy back into an upright position. Perhaps the catch phrase used to market the toy states it best: "Weebles wobble, but they don't fall down." The same quality can apply to people. Just as the Weeble is grounded by a weight, human beings are grounded by their values, relationships, and goals, enabling them to bounce back and remain balanced, no matter how many times they have been knocked down.

Revitalize Your Career

To remain relevant, you may need to refresh or revitalize your career. Think about it in terms of giving your house a facelift by painting your walls a new color, replacing window treatments and floor coverings, or buying new appliances or furniture. If you have ever done that, remember how happy and refreshed you felt afterward. The house was the same, but you gave it new life. That same principle may need to be applied to your career.

A good example of someone who revitalized his career is singer and former teen idol from the 1950s and 1960s, Bobby Rydell. With the British Invasion led by The Beatles in 1964, Bobby's popularity began to wane along with his fellow teen heartthrobs. Although he continued to perform and record, it was never quite the same. His career derailment was exacerbated by several personal challenges in his 60s. The death of his wife, Camille, after a long battle with breast cancer, took its toll. This led to alcohol abuse and major health problems that resulted in a double organ transplant of his liver and kidney and a double heart bypass. Following his surgeries in 2013, he returned to the stage, performing solo to sold-out audiences and frequently appearing with his childhood pals and fellow teen idols, Frankie Avalon and Fabian, in a stage production billed as "The Golden Boys," from 1985 until Bobby's death from pneumonia in April 2022 at age 79. Although his focus was still the songs that made him famous and popular, Bobby refreshed his performances by expanding his repertoire with numbers from the "The Great American Songbook" composers Cole Porter, Irving Berlin, Richard Rogers, and others. He also used technology to enhance his shows with video clips, including the opening scenes from the 2018 Oscar-winning film, *The Green Book,* in which Bobby is portrayed by actor Von Lewis. When asked when how much longer he was going to perform, he answered, "As long as my voice holds up. After all, what would I do? It's all I've known since I was seven years old." Bobby was scheduled to perform at the Golden Nugget Hotel & Casino in Atlantic City in June 2022.

If your career is in a slump, but you're not ready to call it quits, revitalize and refresh it by implementing some of the tips and techniques described in this book. In particular, apply the steps in the reinvention process to your situation.

If and When You Choose to "Retire"

If and when you choose to step away from a paying job, don't *retire*. After all, there is only so much golf you can play, book clubs, garden clubs, and bridge clubs you can join. As Patti and Milledge Hart emphasize throughout their book *The Resolutionist*, you can still add value to society in the post-career phase of your life. In our society, money tends to be the measurement of success and value, but it is not the only measurement. As Stan Silverman, founder and CEO of Silverman Leadership, wrote in his article, "In Retirement, Engage the World in a Different Way" for the *Philadelphia Business Journal*, "Everyone is different. Some people will be happy pursuing a life of leisure after they retire, while others will pursue second careers. Many will pursue an interest that makes a difference in their lives or in the lives of others. One should think where along the retirement continuum they want to be and do what makes them happy and content."

Follow your passion in your post-work phase by using your knowledge and experience to help others. You probably have become less involved or stepped away completely from your participation in professional organizations. Although the organizations may no longer be relevant to your life as they once were, your knowledge and experience are still relevant and can be applied in many situations.

Pro Bono, performing professional services without pay, is most closely associated with the legal profession. However, it can apply to other professions as well. For example, I am doing work pro bono when I conduct seminars and workshops for Providence Animal Center.

Volunteer Involvement

A good example of post-career volunteer involvement where he is applying his professional skills is U.S. Army (retired) Major General Wesley Craig. General Craig began his military career by joining the R.O.T.C. in college during the mid-60s. After graduating from college, he was on active duty for two years followed by 40 years in the Pennsylvania National Guard. He rose through the ranks to become Division Commander from which he retired the first time in 2006. He continued to support the military services as a civilian. He served as Pennsylvania's State Chairman for the Employer Support of the Guard and Reserve, Chairman for the Liberty USO of Pennsylvania and New Jersey, and a member of the United States Army War College Foundation Board of Directors. General Craig was recalled to active service in 2011 as the Adjutant General of Pennsylvania, retiring a second time in 2015.

His impressive military career along with his 32-year career in retail management with the former Strawbridge and Clothier department store in Philadelphia enabled him to develop leadership, financial, and communication skills that he has transferred to his many volunteer responsibilities. In addition to those mentioned, he is active in the Armed Services Council of the Union League of Philadelphia. One of the skills sets he has used in his military-related volunteer work is his ability to supervise and oversee building renovation projects, first for the National Guard alumni group museum and then the renovation of an American Legion building. General Craig remains relevant by continuing to serve and contributing to make things better. He plans on doing so for as long as he can. As he shared during our interview, "If you have abilities, you should use them to help others."

This commitment to helping others is a common theme among all the people I interviewed and is central to remaining relevant. All are philanthropists dedicated to making a difference in the world. Philanthropy is most closely associated with donating large sums of money. While it is true that without the generosity of financial contributors, nonprofits would cease to exist, we cannot and should not overlook or diminish the contributions of people's time and talents for the welfare of our society.

Take Action!

- Create a vision board and display it where you can see it every day.
- Volunteer your professional skills for a cause or organization close to your heart.
- Write one goal for the next phase of your life.

Afterword

Remaining Relevant has been quite a journey. The road to publication has had its share of potholes and detours (medical, personal, financial, and Covid-19). Along the way, I have had to mobilize my internal Global Positioning System (GPS) and roadside assistance: perseverance and resilience.

The three-year journey has been energizing, educational, and enlightening. Taking on this project has been exciting and energizing from the moment I conceived it. It has given me a purpose and a commitment to remain relevant and inspire others to do the same. It has also been very educational. I have learned so much from my research and from my interviews with such incredible and talented people. Finally, it has been enlightening by providing personal insight into and a better understanding of the challenges and changes people face as they age. Nobody really prepares us for getting older.

One major theme emerged from my interviews and can be summarized in two words: passion and purpose. Many of the people I interviewed mentioned the importance of loving what you do along with having a purpose. Think about what makes you want to get out of bed in the morning. Do you love what you do? Do you have a purpose? If so, why retire? As for me, I look to the words of poet Robert Frost from "Stopping by Woods on a Snowy Evening" for inspiration and direction:

"…I have promises to keep, And miles to go before I sleep. And miles to go before I sleep."

References

Bruschi, P. 2003. *Mind Aerobics: The FundaMENTALS of Memory Fitness.* Revised Edition. Yardville, NJ: A MIND AEROBICS publication.

Bruschi, P. 2004. *Quick Tips, Quips and Quotes to Improve Your Mind and Memory.* Yardville, NJ: A MIND AEROBICS publication.

Mehrabian, A. 1980. *Silent Messages: Implicit Communication of Emotions and Attitudes.* 2nd ed. Belmont, CA: Wadsworth Publishing Company.

About the Author

Dr. Karen Lawson is an international consultant, speaker, and author. As founder and president of Lawson Consulting Group, she has built a successful consulting firm specializing in organization and management development as well as executive coaching. She has extensive consulting and seminar experience in the areas of team development, communication, leadership, and quality service across a wide range of industries. Clients include a variety of prominent organizations from financial services, pharmaceutical, telecommunications, manufacturing, health care, government, and education. In her consulting work with Fortune 500 companies as well as small businesses, she uses her experience and knowledge of human interaction to help leaders at all levels make a difference in their organizations.

Karen is the author of 15 books: *The Trainer's Handbook of Leadership Development; The Art of Influencing; Improving On-the-Job Training and Coaching; Improving Performance Through Coaching; The Trainer's Handbook (4 editions); Train-the-Trainer Facilitator's Guide; Involving Your Audience—Making It Active; Skill Builders: 50 Communication Activities; New Employee Orientation Training; Real-World Career Tactics for Women; Leadership Development Basics; Training During Tough Times; 101 Ways to Make Training Active* (co-author). She has also written chapters for 15 different professional collections, in addition to numerous articles in professional journals.

She holds a Doctor of Philosophy degree in Adult and Organization Development from Temple University; a Master of Arts in English from the University of Akron; and a Bachelor of Arts from Mount Union College. She is also a graduate of the National School of Banking in Fairfield, CT. She is one of only 400 people worldwide to have earned the Certified Speaking Professional designation from the 4,000-member National Speakers Association. She has received numerous awards for her outstanding contribution to the training and speaking professions and was also named one of Pennsylvania's "Best 50 Women in Business" as well as one of the *Philadelphia Business Journal's* "Women of Distinction." She also currently serves as Honorary Consul of Fiji for the Commonwealth of Pennsylvania.

She has been actively involved in professional organizations such as the National Speakers Association and the Association for Talent Development, holding leadership positions at both the local and national levels. She is also an active member of the Union League of Philadelphia, Pennsylvania.

Karen is currently an adjunct professor at DeSales University in its MBA programs and has served on the adjunct faculty for Arcadia University, University of Delaware, Saint Joseph's University, Villanova University, Cabrini College, and Rochester Institute of Technology at both the graduate and undergraduate levels. In addition, she conducts online programs for the United Nations System Staff College. She has presented at several professional conferences in the United States, Asia, and Europe.

Index

OTHER TITLES IN THE BUSINESS CAREER DEVELOPMENT COLLECTION

Vilma Barr, Consultant, Editor

- *Pay Attention!* by Cassandra Bailey and Dana M. Schmidt
- *Social Media is About People* by Cassandra Bailey
- *Burn Ladders. Build Bridges.* by Alan M. Patterson
- *Decoding Your STEM Career* by Peter Devenyi
- *A Networking Playbook* by Darryl Howes
- *The Street-Smart Side of Business* by Tara Acosta
- *Rules Don't Work for Me* by Gail Summers
- *Fast Forward Your Career* by Simonetta Lureti and Lucio Furlani
- *Shaping Your Future* by Rita Rocker
- *Emotional Intelligence at Work* by Richard M. Contino and Penelope J. Holt
- *How to Use Marketing Techniques to Get a Great Job* by Edward Barr
- *Negotiate Your Way to Success* by Kasia Jagodzinska
- *How to Make Good Business Decisions* by J.C. Baker
- *Ask the Right Questions; Get the Right Job* by Edward Barr
- *Personal and Career Development* by Claudio A. Rivera and Elza Priede
- *Your GPS to Employment Success* by Beverly A. Williams
- *100 Skills of the Successful Sales Professional* by Alex Dripchak
- *Getting It Right When It Matters Most* by Tony Gambill and Scott Carbonara

Concise and Applied Business Books

The Collection listed above is one of 30 business subject collections that Business Expert Press has grown to make BEP a premiere publisher of print and digital books. Our concise and applied books are for...

- Professionals and Practitioners
- Faculty who adopt our books for courses
- Librarians who know that BEP's Digital Libraries are a unique way to offer students ebooks to download, not restricted with any digital rights management
- Executive Training Course Leaders
- Business Seminar Organizers

Business Expert Press books are for anyone who needs to dig deeper on business ideas, goals, and solutions to everyday problems. Whether one print book, one ebook, or buying a digital library of 110 ebooks, we remain the affordable and smart way to be business smart. For more information, please visit www.businessexpertpress.com, or contact sales@businessexpertpress.com.

CPSIA information can be obtained
at www.ICGtesting.com
Printed in the USA
BVHW050042060123
655682BV00007B/145